Daniel

By the same author

"What Can I Give Him Today?"
– a recipe booklet.

DIANA WELLS

Daniel

Living With An Allergic Child

ASHGROVE PRESS, BATH

First published in Great Britain by
ASHGROVE PRESS LIMITED
19 Circus Place, Bath, Avon BA1 2PW

First published 1985

ISBN 0 906798 61 2 (case)
ISBN 0 906798 62 0 (paper)

Photoset in 11/12½ Palatino by
Ann Buchan (Typesetters)
Walton-on-Thames, Surrey
Printed in Great Britain

Diana Wells S.R.N., R.S.C.N., H.V. cert

Diana Wells trained as a State Registered Nurse and a Sick Children's Nurse in Bristol between 1968 and 1972. After getting married and moving to North Yorkshire she trained as a health visitor and then worked with a busy General Practice just outside York, until Daniel was born in May 1979. Her second son, Jeremy was born in 1980 and the family now lives in Gloucestershire.

In 1983 Diana Wells produced a recipe booklet called "What Can I Give Him Today?", for children allergic to milk, egg and artificial additives. She maintains close contact with the Hyperactive Children's Support Group, and acts as a local contact for families coping with the difficulties of children who have allergies and hyper-sensitivities to foods.

Acknowledgements

I would like to thank Mrs Sandy Austin for the hard work she put into typing my manuscript, and the friends who gave me the initial encouragement to write *Daniel*.

Robert and I will always be grateful for the help and support given to us, in the early years, by my parents. Finally, without Robert's continued love, strength and understanding none of this would have been possible.

Contents

INTRODUCTION

Living with an allergic child can impose a terrific strain on the other members of the household, for many reasons. This is a handicap which can be as disabling initially as many other physical diseases which are well documented and have well established methods of medical treatment. Allergy, however, is so little understood, and is looked on so very sceptically by many doctors, that the family is often left bewildered and with a feeling of total helplessness.

We have lived through these difficulties, but have been more fortunate than many people because we have had a great deal of medical support. Perhaps, because I have trained as a State Registered Nurse and a Health Visitor, I have also had the medical background which has helped me to identify and understand the problems. However, this fact has not insulated us against the crises and traumas that so many families experience.

The purpose of this book is to illustrate the difficulties, the worries, the terrific stress that we as a family have had to cope with, and to show that a positive approach, with an emphasis on self-help, educating the public generally, but also the professionals where possible, is essential.

Having to cope with Daniel's allergies led me to produce a recipe booklet of 50 milk, egg and additive free recipes two years ago, and the interest and response has illustrated the lack of information readily available to the public. The Nursing Times published a short account of the first couple of years of Daniel's problems in May 1982, and this book takes in his first five years: the struggles and the rewards. It includes suggestions for other families coping with allergies, self-help ideas and a new recipe section. A glossary on page 116 explains some of the medical terms used in the book.

9

CHAPTER ONE

Identifying Daniel's Milk Allergy

Daniel was five months old, and normally looked a bonny, fair-haired, blue-eyed baby. However, today his face was swollen, his colour poor, he was covered in large weals and was having difficulty breathing. I had wrapped him in a blanket, and Robert, my husband, was driving us to Casualty. It was tea-time and the roads were busy, and it seemed a very long four miles to our local hospital. Twenty minutes earlier I had started giving Daniel his tea. I had mixed up a savoury powdered baby food with water, and he had just had a taste off the spoon. Almost instantly he started coughing and choking; then urticarial weals appeared around his mouth and neck, and I could see them on his wrists too. He was sick all down his clothes, and I took him out of his chair and started to take off his baby suit. His tummy and legs were producing those red, blistery weals, and he started crying. His eyes were getting very puffy and beginning to close, and his neck was also swelling. His crying began to get very husky, and his colour to deteriorate.

It all happened so quickly, and for all my past nursing experience, I felt alarmed. This was my baby, obviously in an acute allergic state, and I felt helpless. I rang my neighbour, who came over immediately, and I asked her to ring the doctor's surgery for me. The receptionist told her that there was no surgery that evening in the village, but put her through to one of the G.P.s. His advice was to take Daniel immediately to Casualty. He was choking and still trying to be sick. By this time Robert had arrived home, and here we were driving to the hospital.

In the Casualty Department, his condition had not worsened. The doctor examined him and asked lots of

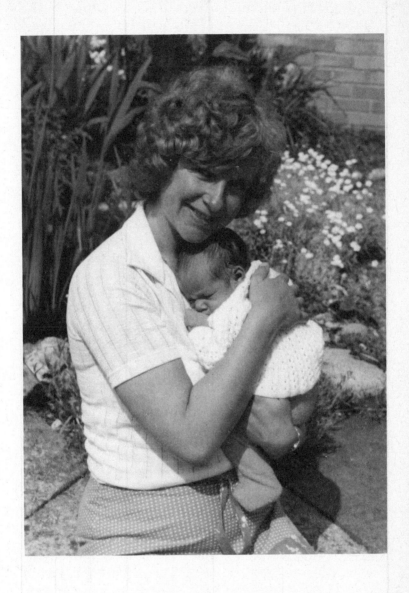

"Daniel was born in May 1979"

questions, and stated the obvious. It was an allergy and he suspected cow's milk: one of the ingredients of the baby food. He wrote a letter for our G.P. which we had to deliver, and was happy that we should take Daniel home.

Daniel was born in May 1979. I had an uneventful pregnancy and a normal delivery, and he was an alert, responsive 8lb baby. We stayed in the maternity hospital for eight days and he was pronounced fit and healthy on discharge. However, over the next three or four weeks he developed an angry, blistery rash on his face. He was very irritable and constantly rubbing his face, either on his carry cot sheet or on me, if I was cuddling him. Our G.P. suspected infantile eczema and prescribed an ointment to smooth on the skin, but his irritability and obvious discomfort increased. In despair I took him back to the surgery within twenty-four hours, and on that occasion saw another doctor who diagnosed a staphylococcal skin infection, and accordingly prescribed antibiotics. The response was dramatic and his skin cleared quickly. I was breast feeding Daniel on demand, and he was a very thirsty baby, taking eight or nine feeds a day, with drinks of boiled water in between. He was always restless and during the day slept very little. An hour at any one time would be a good sleep for Daniel, then as long as he was cuddled he would be fairly content.

By the time he was about six weeks old his skin had a very "tough", scaly appearance, and we were advised to bath him as infrequently as possible, using oilatum in the bath rather than soap when we did. I also noticed that each time I breast fed him his skin developed a rash, over his trunk and face. By the next feed this rash had disappeared but would reappear by the end of the feed. His stools were absolutely explosive, soaking through his nappy and clothes, and going right through my skirts and petticoats too. I used to have to shower and change if he had been sitting on my knee when he had his bowels open.

At about this time I read an article in the *Health Visitor* about the possibility of cow's milk allergy showing in an infant who was being breast fed. I decided to eliminate all cow's milk products from my diet for a trial period to see whether this had any effect on Daniel. Robert was away in France for ten days, so I did not have to worry about his food. I cancelled our milk order, ate no cheese, butter, chocolate, ice cream etc., and within a week the rash had totally disappeared. Daniel's stools had returned to the "normal" breast-fed baby stools, and I seriously wondered whether a cow's milk allergy was possible. My doctor discounted it totally, dismissing any possibility of such an allergy showing through the breast milk. He explained to me that the protein in my diet would be considerably altered by the time its nutrients were transferred through my breast milk to Daniel, consequently it was not feasible to be thinking in terms of cow's milk allergy in such a young infant. This, coupled with the fact that there was no history of allergy in the form of eczema, asthma or hayfever in either my family or Robert's reduced the possibility even further. I was not convinced by his argument and explained where I had read the article, but he was unimpressed. I, however, had seen the results of my experiment, and was very concerned about the possible consequences, as I was sure that there was a sensitivity to milk protein.

When Daniel was three months old we went over to Dublin for a holiday with my brother, who was living and working there at the time. My memories of this holiday are overshadowed by Daniel's constant crying. All he seemed to do was cry and feed. I can remember being very tearful myself, as I was so tired by the repeated nightly routine of being up at least three times during the night for feeds. It was never a quick suck and tuck up again, as he always filled his nappy, which usually required a change of nightie as well; and then he was up for good by about 5.30 a.m. I was beginning to wonder when he would let us sleep through the night. Little did I know at that stage!

He had his first immunization. I had read the Government guidelines on immunization and the contra-indications to the whooping-cough vaccine, and had noted that allergy was not a contra-indication. I had seen many babies with the disease, and Robert and I discussed it at length. We wanted him to have the triple vaccine. My doctor was happy to do it; and I will admit that we were anxious for twenty-four hours, but there was no reaction. We were pleased that that hurdle was over.

At about four months I felt Daniel was needing more than just breast milk so I started to introduce a taste at a time of puréed food. Initially I gave him apple and baby rice. He enjoyed them and I hoped that being a little more satisfied he might sleep longer than about three hours at a time during the night. Unfortunately, it made no difference. One day I tried him with a powdered baby food, mixed with boiled water, and on that occasion noticed weals appearing around his mouth, spreading to his neck. It occurred to me that I had perhaps been a little heavy handed with his spoon, mopping up the dribbles around his chin. As he was totally unconcerned I thought little more about it. It was about a month later when the episode occurred which resulted in our visit to Casualty. I had only given him "home cooking": i.e. puréed vegetables and fruit, in between those two occasions, and he had therefore had no other contact with any milk product.

I asked my G.P. if we could be referred to a paediatrician, as I felt that Daniel had a potentially serious problem, which we seemed to be having to cope with totally on our own. I needed confirmation, and also advice for the future. As a practising Health Visitor I had had contact with babies who had milk allergy, but symptoms can vary so much from infant to infant. They may be as diverse as persistent colic, eczema, wheezing attacks, loose stools, failure to thrive, severe cradle cap, very sore buttocks, etc., and parents and doctors try all the usual remedies in an effort to sort out the problems; but inevitably with no success. It seems very hard to accept that a food as "natural and healthy" as milk could possibly be the cause of so much misery and ill-health for the affected child.

The paediatrician from the local hospital visited us at home one Saturday morning. He examined Daniel thoroughly, and of course he looked the picture of health, beaming at him from the rug on the floor. He took a very detailed history, and confirmed that Daniel had displayed the characteristic signs of cow's milk allergy. He reassured us that many babies have this sort of problem due to their immature immune system, but that by the time they are eighteen months old they have usually grown out of it and can eat a normal diet again. He advised a diet totally devoid of milk or any milk products, also egg and fish, as these proteins often caused similar problems in children displaying a cow's milk allergy. He advised that I should breast feed for as long as I could, but that then I should give Nutramigen, obtained on prescription, as a milk substitute. He also arranged for me to see a dietitian and lent me a book which contained a chapter on food allergies in infants. It was highly technical and much of it was beyond my understanding; nevertheless it gave us a little more insight into the problem. He suggested to us that when Daniel was about eighteen months old that he should admit him to the children's ward, in order to challenge him with milk. This way, if there were going to be any problems, then he was obviously in the right place for immediate treatment.

The next few months were uneventful. Daniel's second immunization was given with no ill-effect. The only other allergic reaction he had was after he had eaten a liquidized bacon and tomato mixture. When I changed his nappy he had erupted in angry, red blistery weals again, this time from his knees to his waist. They disappeared after a couple of hours, causing no more discomfort than an obvious irritation to him. I mentally stored away the suspect food (tomatoes); not to be given again for quite a long time.

I had confirmation of a second pregnancy when Daniel was seven months old. We had decided to have two children close together, and obviously at that time had no idea what problems were going to present themselves in the future, or I am sure we would not have considered having another child so quickly. Our nights were still very broken, but we felt they could only get better, and that now

Daniel

Daniel was much more active and crawling everywhere, he was bound to sleep better. He enjoyed his food and used to eat Weetabix with Ribena on it for breakfast, or porridge made with water. We had made our own bread before Daniel was born, so to continue with this practice was no hardship, and the more practice we had, the better the results. The dietitian had informed us that many commercially prepared loaves contained milk products in one form or another, so home baking was safer. I tried making custard with Nutramigen, but the taste and smell were very strong and Daniel was not interested at all. He readily adapted to drinking Nutramigen, but would not tolerate it used in cooking, or on his cereal. I found his diet rather limiting and repetitive. It would have been convenient and easy to give him a boiled egg or cheese fingers, but we seemed to provide him with acceptable alternatives: I puréed meat and vegetable combinations; he enjoyed chicken, and I made jellies or gave him mashed banana and other fruits for desserts. I searched the shelves in food shops, avidly reading ingredients on food jars and packets. The number of baby food preparations that didn't contain skimmed milk powder, whey, caseinates, egg, etc, were few and far between. In the end I found it easier to cook and freeze small amounts, when I was absolutely sure of the contents of the food.

Our surgery in the village had its own pharmacy, so I used to collect two or three tins of Nutramigen at a time from them. The Nutramigen powder is made up like any other baby milk powder, but only one scoop of powder is used to two ounces of water. It is very difficult to mix, and I whisk it to obtain a less lumpy mixture, and then very often sieve it too. It is a complete food in itself, containing all the necessary minerals, vitamins, fats and protein, so I felt reassured that Daniel's diet in combination with Nutramigen was well balanced and nutritious. He certainly did not look as if he was failing to thrive. His skin was clear and healthy, his weight increasing in proportion to his height. He had gained his milestones within normal limits, and was producing strong, healthy teeth. He had had a couple

16

of ear infections and a viral infection which caused sickness and a widespread rash, but otherwise had remained fairly healthy. His stools were still loose, even though he was no longer breast-fed. His skin had lost the roughness and scaly quality it had had earlier, and we stopped using oilatum and began to use soap and to bath him more frequently.

As his motor development increased, so his exploring and climbing activities increased. I had to have an eye on him at all times. He was into every cupboard, onto every shelf he could climb onto, constantly into scrapes. I remember my parents coming to stay on one occasion and my mother saying, "When do you ever do any work?" "What do you mean?" I asked, and she said I never seemed to have a minutes rest as I was always pulling him out of cupboards, replacing books on the bookshelves that he had scattered everywhere, removing the phone from him, lifting him down from tables and the backs of chairs, rescuing him from one scrape after another. He was not a child who would sit in his high chair and be amused for ten minutes. He cried and had terrible screaming bouts if he was restricted in any way, and I found I had to go out for long walks, regardless of weather or fatigue, just to try to get him to sleep for half an hour. At night he was still up several times, and always awake very early. I tried everything I could think of to keep him amused in the morning: plenty of activities in his cot, warmer room, music to listen to, but there was absolutely no way he was going to stay in his cot, or for that matter let anyone else sleep if he wasn't going to. He gnawed the top of his cot to pieces, he screamed, he cried, he shouted, and no amount of ignoring him, pacifying him or bribing him made any difference whatsoever. In the end I decided it was easier to get up, get him up and at least have a quieter household.

At about this time, we found that we were going to move house, from Yorkshire down to Warwickshire. We put our house on the market and sold it very quickly, so we had to find a house quickly too. The first weekend we went house hunting we stayed with relatives. Daniel would not settle our first night there. He cried and screamed, and at one o'clock in the morning I had packed our suitcases and told the long suffering relatives that we were going to leave. They persuaded us to let Daniel run around downstairs while we all had a cup of tea, and eventually he wore himself out and we managed to get four or five hours sleep. Going away was something of a mammoth task, as besides all the necessary equipment one needs for a one-year-old we had to ensure that we had enough suitable food as well. We were worn to a frazzle at the end of our first day. In and out of the car, in and out of people's homes, and Daniel had screamed and cried and fought. He hadn't slept at all. He was exhausted and fractious, and we decided to go home.

A future colleague had generously offered us accommodation the following weekend, where we would be more local for our house hunting. We gratefully accepted his hospitality. Again Daniel was extremely difficult to settle and I was anxious and tired and very pregnant, but we had a successful weekend. Our hosts were marvellous. They said they had never been up so early in the morning! But they took it all in their stride. On the Sunday morning we were chatting over breakfast and Daniel was playing round the house and in and out of the garden. It was a lovely warm sunny day. He bounced in and caught my arm, just as I was finishing a rather cold cup of tea, and some of the tea splashed on his jumper. I mopped it up, but then thought I'd take off his jumper and rinse it, as half an hour on the line in the sunshine would dry it. Within a couple of minutes of taking the jumper off Robert said, "What's Daniel done to his arm?" It was swelling with urticarial weals, large, red and white blistery weals. Where the tea had soaked through his jumper he was reacting, presumably to the milk. That was the first time we had seen a reaction of that nature, and I had certainly never come across anyone reacting to skin contact like that.

It was obviously itchy and he scratched it as it irritated him, but the reaction had disappeared by lunch time. I was rather worried, as Daniel had completely avoided any milk or milk products, and having had no reactions since our

18

visit to Casualty, we were rather assuming that he was "growing out of it" as the paediatrician had suggested.

The next time I saw my G.P. was to inform her that we were moving shortly, and to ask if we could take a letter to our new G.P. informing him of Daniel's problems, and explaining that we required regular prescriptions for Nutramigen. I told her about the incident with the spilt tea, and she was duly concerned: but other than mentioning it in her letter, felt she really could do nothing more as we were moving. She checked on Daniel's immunization programme, which was up to date. He had completed the third injection and we had been advised not to have the measles vaccine because it is cultured on egg and could therefore invoke an allergic response if given to someone who is sensitive to egg protein.

We actually moved house within six weeks of putting our house on the market. It was a hectic time and looking back it is difficult to see how we organised ourselves. Daniel was as energetic and lively as ever. I remember a friend calling one day and I was in the kitchen feeling more than a little flustered. I had arranged every chair we possessed around all the kitchen units. "Whatever are you doing?" she asked. "I'm trying to keep Daniel out of the cupboards – as fast as I remove him from one, he's into the next". While he found the chairs quite an effective barricade, he then climbed on top, so that nothing was safe on top of the units. All our packing had to be done when Daniel was in bed, or at weekends when one of us could remove him from the scene and let the other make some progress.

He was just thirteen months when we moved, not quite walking independently, but walking around the furniture, and he could move like lightning. He had a whale of a time "helping" to unpack, exploring all the rooms and garden. My parents came to stay for a few days, and it was really only with their help that we managed to get organised quickly. Daniel didn't settle at night, but then he had had a lot to cope with: change in routine, stress attached to the move, new addition to the family imminent and he was

Daniel

cutting teeth. With all these problems we could hardly expect him to adapt to our new home immediately.

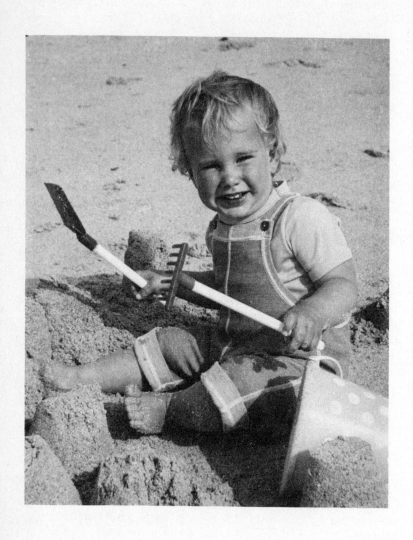

Daniel aged one, clearly thriving on his restricted diet

CHAPTER TWO

Daniel's Hyperactivity

I had had a busy morning. The new baby was due in just over two weeks and I had been baking cakes, bread and pies for the freezer. My parents were coming to stay when I went into hospital, and I wanted as much preparation done in advance as possible. I sat down on the settee feeling quite weary. Daniel jumped up on my knee with a book. He decided to sit one side of me, then the other, and climbed over my cumbersome frame while he was making up his mind. With that I felt my waters break, so the next half an hour was spent collecting together last things for my suitcase, ringing hospital and parents, and travelling in to the hospital maternity unit.

Jeremy was born at 1 a.m. that night. We were delighted to have a brother for Daniel, and relieved that all had gone smoothly. Unfortunately problems occurred the next day as Jeremy developed a hole in his lung, and for the next ten days he was kept in the Special Care Baby Unit. Initially he was tube fed, and I insisted that absolutely no cow's milk should be given, explaining about Daniel's problems. He was given expressed breast milk when possible, and topped up with soya milk. The paediatrician enquired about Daniel and I was pleased to have an opportunity to talk to him, although I would obviously have preferred somewhat different circumstances. He was not unduly concerned about the milk allergy, stating that it would almost certainly have disappeared by eighteen months to two years. He suggested that I did a very small challenge at home, nearer the time. I was rather perturbed by his attitude, but decided to ignore that for the time being and concentrate on Jeremy's problems.

Straight after birth, Jeremy had been taken to Special

Care, partly because of the time of night, and partly because he was rather snuffly. During the next day the nursing staff had kept me informed of his progress but hadn't brought him down to see me because they said he was having difficulty maintaining his temperature. He had also become hypoglycaemic and would not suck when they had tried to give him glucose water, so they had put a naso-gastric tube down. They helped me to express colostrum and assured me that they would bring him down for visiting at 3 o'clock. A Special Care nurse brought him and allowed him to stay for five minutes, but then whisked him back up to the Unit. After my visitors had gone, I went up to the Special Care Unit for the first time, and was encouraged to cuddle him and attempted to feed him. It was while I was doing this that he suddenly went blue. He was immediately placed in oxygen in an incubator, and the paediatrician was called. X-rays revealed a spontaneous pneumo-mediastinum causing respiratory difficulties, and also embarrassing his heart rate. I was told that he had produced a hole in his lung which had allowed air to escape and this had gone into the cavity in which the heart lay.

The next few days were emotionally draining, but the nursing and medical staff were very helpful and understanding, and I was reassured by their constant attention and explanations of what was happening. Robert visited me every afternoon and evening. Being a teacher, he was on school summer holiday. He brought Daniel during the afternoons, but usually let him run around outside with one of my parents. The first day when he brought him in he had been into everyone else's locker, under all the beds, and generally caused some confusion. He had disliked being restrained and had struggled and screamed, so we felt it best that I should be allowed to see him running around outside, but not let him run riot in the ward.

Jeremy made steady progress. His condition gradually improved and by his eighth day he was taking a 3oz feed from me, so his tube was removed. He had lost 14oz in weight, but as over the next two days he started to regain weight, I was allowed to take him home on the eleventh day.

I expected problems with Daniel, but on the whole he accepted both me and Jeremy very well. He was rather off-hand with me initially, but soon showed affection and interest in Jeremy. I gave him as much attention as I could over the next few weeks, and was agreeably surprised at his apparent adjustment to our new family member. The most fraught times were when I was feeding Jeremy, and I had to have every trick I could think of up my sleeve to hold his attention. I read or sang to him, made up stories and tried to have his favourite playthings readily to hand. He was easily distracted and inevitably ended up by getting into mischief which meant interrupting Jeremy's feed to sort him out.

Daniel had been walking a couple of months now and this extra freedom gave him new outlets for his energy. He didn't sit down very much at all. At meal times he was strapped into his chair, and after his lunch I did manage to get him to sleep for about half an hour. This allowed me to recharge my batteries, and also think about preparing our evening meal. I had to use those quiet moments to do the various activities which were quite impossible when Daniel was up. He was a voluble child, even though he had no words. He screamed and shouted and cried. He used to lie on the floor kicking the doors or wall if I wanted him to do something that he didn't. Night times were dreadful. We could get him to bed by about six o'clock and he usually went straight to sleep until about ten o'clock. Then he woke and cried and just seemed to want to drink and drink. He would not settle for any length of time then, and we were in and out of his bedroom for the rest of the night. The amount he was drinking was causing wet beds and pyjamas, even though he wore a double terry nappy. The screaming was inevitable. It happened every night whatever we did. We tried very firm handling, ignoring it, cuddling and lots of attention, night lights, musical boxes, food, sedation. We tried everything we could think of, but either Daniel had got into a rut with this behaviour or else

23

there was a problem which completely baffled us. As soon as the noise started one or other of us ran in to try and stop it. We were worried that we were annoying neighbours, and anxious that we shouldn't start waking Jeremy in the same vein, every night. It was a vicious circle, and we became quite exhausted. I of course was also up to give Jeremy a feed during the night, but he soon dropped the very early morning feed: something Daniel never seemed to do. Jeremy also slept as long as four hours at a time during the day: again, something Daniel never did: and that helped to take the pressure off, a little.

Daniel was also getting rather persistent ear and chest infections, and it seemed to me that about once a fortnight I was having to take him to the surgery where he usually ended up on a course of antibiotics. One day he was particularly fractious. I had taken him to the doctor that morning, and he had tonsillitis and a middle ear infection, so I put his behaviour down to being poorly, and tried to give him extra cuddles and attention: which he usually resisted. He would not eat or drink: most unusual to refuse fluids, and then I noticed a nasty, blistery rash on the palms of his hands, on his knees, and also over his buttocks when I changed his nappy. I rang my Health Visitor who called in to see him. She suggested that he might have a streptococcal rash, as a result of his throat infection, but as he was on antibiotics, not to worry too much. That afternoon I could not pacify him. He cried and screamed and fought, and by tea-time I felt exhausted. I noticed at this time that he was also dribbling all the time. He seemed unable to swallow his saliva. I spoke to our G.P. on the phone and he popped in to see him after surgery.

Daniel had hand, foot and mouth disease. Apparently there had been quite an epidemic in the area some months before, and Daniel had contracted it somehow. I felt I knew where. The previous day I had taken him to buy a pair of shoes. Needless to say, he had been up to all sorts of mischief in the shoe shop, and on one occasion I found him behind a shelf with the shoe horn in his mouth. His mouth was covered in ulcers, all over his tongue, soft and hard palate, and inside his cheeks. It was no wonder he was so miserable. The doctor advised me to give him ¼ disprin tablet every four hours during the day and night.

The next few days and nights were a nightmare. Daniel's behaviour just had to be seen to be believed. He cried and screamed incessantly. He was irritable, aggressive and unco-operative. He snatched about 30 minutes sleep, then woke fretful and restless. He wanted one of us with him constantly, but would not be cuddled or pacified. He would not lie down with us, or let us rest either. The disprin did not seem to relieve his obvious discomfort, but rather to increase his irritability, although at the time I was too worried and tired to be able to see this. Jeremy survived with the bare essentials that week. He was fed and changed, topped and tailed. I was so relieved that he would sleep, and was contented between feeds. As Daniel's mouth ulcers improved, so I tailed off the disprin, and the general misery and irritability gradually disappeared, and once again Daniel was back to his usual noisy, energetic self.

During Jeremy's first few months I used to go to the clinic every couple of weeks, partly as a social activity, and partly to keep a check on Jeremy, as he had had rather a rough start in life. I used to look at the other mothers there, often with a child sitting quietly on a chair to one side, while they cuddled a new baby. Then I would look at Daniel as he charged around the clinic, in and out of the rooms, up and down the slide, on and off the rocking horse. It made me feel tired just to watch him.

Any trip out became a major expedition, whether it was shopping or visiting a friend; even going to the surgery. In the first instance I had to battle even to get Daniel to sit on the pram seat. He used to arch his back, try to stand on the pram, cry and kick me. Every mother knows the hostile stares of uninformed passers-by as they mutter about unmanageable children. If I relented and let him run, on his reins, he resented the restriction, and usually ended up by lying screaming in the road.

I had – I hoped, unobtrusively – stopped visiting some

25

friends as Daniel's behaviour was not very sociable. He couldn't help diving into all their nooks and crannies, emptying drawers, fiddling with their trinkets and generally producing chaos within a short stay. Books were removed from bookcases, entire toy collections dispersed through the house, boxes of jig-saws and games emptied in a pile on the floor, telephones constantly tampered with. He flitted from one scene of destruction to another, unable to sit still and concentrate on one activity. I spent the whole time apologising, making excuses and feeling thoroughly embarrassed. I am sure there was a great sigh of relief after we had all gone home. It was the same at our house. Daniel destroyed any make believe play or games other children were playing at. His constant attention-seeking and crying, displays of frustration and aggression and general antisocial behaviour were not conducive to entertaining friends. I preferred to go out in the garden and let Daniel run off his energies there, or visit the local park where he could swing and climb and shout without offending anyone else.

Many times we asked ourselves why we should have produced a child like this. Here we were, two parents who were well educated; well informed on child rearing, attitudes to management and discipline etc. I, particularly, was very used to dealing with infants and toddlers. Our marriage was stable. We had a happy home environment – admittedly not terribly relaxed and free from stress – but nevertheless, not coping with major social problems such as unemployment or poor housing: and yet, still we seemed to be producing a child who was causing so many headaches for us. Where were we going wrong?

Daniel still wasn't saying anything, although he was about 18 months old now, but his comprehension was excellent. He communicated his feelings and wants excellently, and I suppose, because we understood, he didn't have to make too much effort to talk. I wasn't terribly concerned about his speech because he obviously heard and understood. He was still constantly getting infections and, because we were so tired, I asked if we could have some sedation to give him, just now and again, so that we could get some sleep. I used it in desperation really, because it didn't seem to help much. He may have slept for about four hours at a time, but that was only when we gave double or triple the dose, and then the next morning he seemed more excitable than ever. It really was not worth it. It was just a straw we clung to.

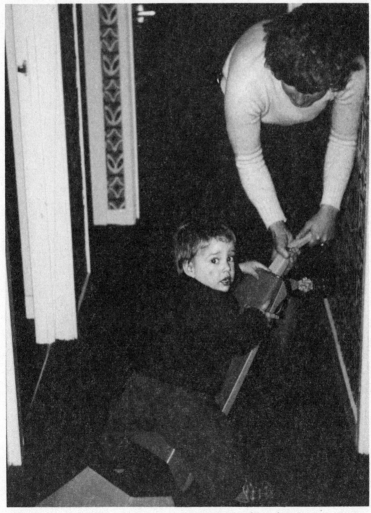

How do you ever manage to get anything done?

CHAPTER THREE

A Diet to Reduce Hyperactivity

December 1980 was not a good month for Jeremy. He was just 3½ months old, and had a chest infection which would not clear. He coughed and coughed, was not interested in feeding and was sleeping badly at night. He started to wheeze too, which rather worried me. None of the decongestants and antibiotics he had improved the situation. Christmas Day was very quiet. Both boys had bronchitis and were alternately fractious, and then would sleep for a while. We didn't have any visitors and didn't feel we could take the boys very far either. On December 28th Jeremy was christened and friends and relatives came to spend the day with us. He was wrapped up in shawls and blankets to keep him warm. Daniel had to be taken into the crèche by my Mother, as he was intent on wrecking the Nativity Scene up by the altar and could not be persuaded to look at books, or play with any of the activities we had taken for him. Phyl, a close nursing friend of mine, was Jeremy's godmother, and I remember her disappearing with him, as soon as we got back to the house, to give him an intensive chest phsyiotherapy session! The following day the doctor admitted him to hospital for observation and chest X-ray. I stayed with him in the mother and baby unit for about three days. The doctors said there was nothing seriously wrong, and that the wheezing would gradually disappear.

Because Daniel's behaviour at night was so bad, I decided to keep a food diary and to record every item of food and drink that he had, with a comment at the end of the day on behaviour etc. I measured his night time consumption of liquid and between 6p.m. and 6a.m. He was often drinking between two and three litres of fluid. It was no wonder we had soaking wet beds and pyjamas. We tried to cut down on the drinks, but this resulted in even more screaming, and in the early hours of the morning one will do anything for peace and quiet.

Another friend had also suggested that we tried removing artificial additives from Daniel's diet, to see whether they had any bearing on his behaviour. She had tried a similar experiment on her child with excellent results. There wasn't much in the way of artificial additives in Daniel's diet, although I did occasionally make jelly, and his favourite drink was blackcurrant juice, which was of course flavoured and coloured. So, one day (we were actually going to my parents for the weekend) I bought some fresh fruit juice, and we decided that Daniel should only drink diluted juice, or Nutramigen; and we carefully monitored all foods. The first night we put him to bed, and could not believe it when when we didn't see him until 6 a.m. the next day. I dashed in, wondering if he was all right, and there he was just waking up. It really seemed far too good to be true: even my parents remarked about his general behaviour. He was quieter, much more amenable, less aggressive, more affectionate. It was difficult to realize that only twenty-four hours had elapsed since we had stopped the blackcurrant drink. For about a week the improvement was maintained, but then he started slipping back into his old pattern of broken nights, temper tantrums etc. However, we had seen the remarkable change, and I was determined to explore those possibilities to the full. I didn't know much about the ingredients of foods, the preservative which prolonged the shelf life, the colours and flavours to excite the eye and palate, but if these were harming Daniel then I wanted as much information as possible. I wrote off to the Hyperactive Children's Support Group, sending a stamped addressed envelope, and eagerly awaited their reply. I wasn't disappointed, and had a lot of information to read and digest. It appeared that besides the additives in food, some foods naturally contain a substance called salicylate. This too can produce the same symptoms as the chemical additives, in a sensitive person. We eliminated foods containing the salicylates from Daniel's diet as well, and once again found that we had a much calmer, more agreeable child. He started to sleep at night again, and friends and relatives remarked about the change in him.

Over the next few weeks we began to feel more human, as we were sleeping well and enjoying each other's company. I firmly believe that if you get a good night's sleep you can cope with whatever the day presents. I had been so weary that my patience was stretched to its limits, and I felt I couldn't be bothered with anything or anyone. I had to make an effort to keep on top of the food preparation because Daniel's milk and egg allergy demanded that most biscuits and all cakes had to be home baked. I had to make pies and bread, and couldn't resort to any convenience foods. In addition the extra strain of no additives meant even more preparation: but we were well motivated. There was no way that we could continue in the same vein as the last two years. The knowledge that salicylates could produce the irritability, aggression and behaviour problems that Daniel displayed, was given greater credibility when I though back on the atrocious behaviour he had shown when I was giving him disprin (disprin contains salicylate). On one other occasion since the hand, foot and mouth infection I had again given him disprin. He was teething, and very miserable, but the next few hours resulted in an exacerbation of his sleep and behaviour problems.

I decided now to ask my Health Visitor's advice about trying a milk challenge. She suggested that I give a tiny piece of cheese, mixed in with Daniel's dinner, rather than a cow's milk trial. I cut a wafer thin morsel of cheese, about half a centimetre square and mixed it in with his meat and potato one day. Within a few minutes there were signs of urticaria appearing again: his sensitivity was obviously still acute.

Shortly after this, some friends came to see us one afternoon, and William, then three years old, asked if he could have a drink of milk. He left his cup on the edge of the table, and I thought no more about it. After they had gone, I saw Daniel reach up and tip the cup towards him to see what was in it. William had left about an ounce of milk, and this trickled onto the bib of Daniel's dungarees. I took him into the bathroom and undressed him, pulling his jumper and vest off too. I washed him with water, and as I did this I could see the red, blistery weals beginning to erupt. From his waist up to his scalp Daniel was soon covered in urticaria. His face swelled up, his eyes became very puffy and almost closed, and he was very miserable. The general swelling gradually subsided, but left him with a blistery rash, particularly bad in the region of his face. This persisted for about a week.

I was really alarmed by this episode and went to see my doctor. I voiced my fears of what I felt might happen if Daniel accidentally drank any milk: that the result could be fatal if medical help was not readily available. She felt this was a distinct possibility. The implications of this began to dawn on me. We would have to be incredibly vigilant in our home, and when we visited friends: far more so than I had ever anticipated. It was a sobering thought that many of the foods which formed our everyday diet were potentially so very harmful to Daniel: milk, butter and margarine, cheese, yoghurt, cakes and biscuits, some cereals, some bread, chocolate, many puddings etc. She said she would refer us to a specialist, but was not sure to which department she should make the referral. She decided on Dermatology at the Birmingham Children's Hospital, and we had an out-patient appointment within about three weeks. On two occasions before we went for this appointment Daniel had conjunctivitis with very swollen eyes. He had been playing in the kitchen and reached up to the draining board, then rubbed his eye. He had obviously touched some water which presumably contained milk from the washing up water, and any contact, particularly in the region of the face, caused instant swelling.

CHAPTER FOUR

A Fortnight In Hospital

The day of our out-patient visit was sunny and warm. A friend offered to come to Birmingham with me, for company, and also so that she could look after Jeremy while I took Daniel into the doctor. Out-patient clinics are notoriously busy, and Daniel had plenty of time to run around, play on the rocking horses and in the Wendy house. Our name was called at last, and we went in to see the Registrar, an Indian lady doctor. She had a letter explaining Daniel's problems, but asked me to tell her the whole story, starting from his first allergic reaction. She said she had not come across a problem quite like Daniel's before, and suggested that he should be admitted for full investigation. She stressed that I must stay with him, especially at meal times, and that I must impress on the ward staff the importance of his diet. On our way out I gave the Admissions Officer all the necessary details, and she said we would be hearing from them in about a month.

About two weeks later Daniel started with sickness and diarrhoea. It came on very suddenly one evening about six o'clock, and continued for the next ten days. He was having diarrhoea up to a dozen times a day, although he was quite well in himself; and, after the initial sickness, felt well enough to eat and drink. The diarrhoea was profuse, and as he was still in nappies it meant that I had a lot of washing. I was talking to a neighbour one day, and she said, "When did Daniel's diarrhoea start?".

"On Monday evening", I replied. "Why?"

"Did you read in the paper last week that the Water Authority would be adding Pyrethrum to the water as from Monday, to kill all the little shrimps etc in the water supply? Apparently they do this every few years".

I decided to ring the relevant department to ask if there could possibly be any reaction as a result of adding this chemical to the water. After about six phone calls and numerous explanations I eventually spoke to someone who was very much on the defensive, and said that it had never been known to affect humans, and was absolutely safe. I tried to explain about Daniel's sensitivities, but he was not willing to concede that there was even the slightest possibility that the water was causing his problems.

The next day we had a phone call from the Sister on Ward 9 at the Children's Hospital asking if we could take Daniel in the following day to start his investigations. She said they would have Nutramigen on the ward, and that the dietitian would sort out his diet with me, so not to worry about food. I rang my parents who were happy to come up and help Robert look after Jeremy, and we told Daniel all about his "adventure". He did not have a particular cuddly toy that was a favourite, but said he would like to take Teddy, so I duly sewed a name tag on, along with labels on his clothes. I must admit that I was a little apprehensive, purely from the food point of view. When I have prepared a meal I know that is is completely safe. But I just had to accept that the food that would be given to Daniel was perfectly all right for him. I was determined not to be the "fussy mother", but on the other hand I was also determined to be very firm about what he could and could not eat.

The next day my parents drove us all to the Hospital and we waved goodbye to them when a porter arrived to take us to the ward. The ward had about sixteen cots and beds, and had a mixture of patients, some with skin diseases and some with infectious illnesses, so many of the children were confined to cubicles. He was shown his cot and locker, and he explored his little room, put Teddy to bed and played with the toys that had been put there for him. He had his own colour television to watch, and the little boy in the next cubicle came in shyly to see who his new neighbour was.

Daniel was weighed and had a name tag put on his wrist.

Daniel

He had a urine bag attached to him to collect a specimen for routine testing, and a nurse took all the basic details down on a form. The dietitian came to see us, and said that all Daniel's meals would be sent up individually from the diet kitchen.

About half an hour later the first tray arrived. It was tea-time. I looked at it in amazement. There was a "mousse" of sorts on the tray. However had they produced that? I had never found a way of making anything look remotely like a mousse! However I was still determined not to be too fussy, so I mentally congratulated the dietitian on her inventiveness. Daniel's face lit up. He had never seen anything like that either, and he tried it first. Instantly he pushed the tray away and put his hand to his mouth. He was obviously very unhappy and started retching, and then vomited all over his clothes and the floor. The staff nurse came in and I suggested that the mousse contained milk. She was quite indignant and said it was Daniel's meal, sent specially from the diet kitchen.

"He is excited and rather nervous about coming into hospital", she said. "The sickness is probably a nervous reaction. He hasn't even eaten half a teaspoon, so it can't possibly be the food".

I explained that it only needed to be a taste to cause a reaction, and that Daniel didn't react by vomiting if he was anxious about a situation. I was sure it was the food. She had cleared up the mess by now, and brought clean clothes for him. I changed him and put him in his cot, as he was so unhappy. His face was scarlet and puffy, and he was holding his tummy. He was sick again, this time all over the cot, and once again the Staff Nurse came in to change the bedclothes. By now Daniel had urticaria around his face and on his arms and legs: in fact where his vomit had splashed down him.

There was no doubt about the food. I was very unhappy: partly because of Daniel's predicament, and partly because this was our first day, first meal in hospital, and my fears were already proving to be very real. It appeared that the "wrong diet" had been given in error. Everyone was extremely apologetic, and whereas no real harm was done, the episode did serve to underline the seriousness of the situation. Daniel was reluctant to eat very much at all during his stay in hospital. I'm sure he was suspicious of the food, and who could blame him? His reactions obviously upset him a great deal.

He still had profuse diarrhoea when he was admitted, but over the first forty-eight hours this gradually subsided and by the third day he was back to his "normal" loose stools which occurred once or twice a day. We were, of course, under a different water authority in Birmingham. I'm not convinced that the Pyrethrum wasn't the cause of all the diarhoea.

Daniel spent most of a fortnight in hospital, and had a variety of tests and investigations. He was seen by many doctors who asked numerous questions, and ultimately we were referred to the Gastroenterology Department. The Registrar came to see me, to introduce himself, and to look at Daniel. While we were talking Daniel emptied a tin of talcum powder all over the doctor's black shoes, and the bottom of his dark suit trousers. I was very embarrassed, but he took it all in good part, and said he had a son about the same age as Daniel, who also got up to all sorts of pranks.

The doctor reassured me by saying he had seen children similiar to Daniel before, and that they all improved, usually by the age of four or five. He said he hadn't seen one with the same severity of reaction reach school age, still reacting so severely. I asked him about trying to desensitize him, but he said this wasn't really feasible. It is apparently much more difficult to desensitize people who are allergic to food than it is to other allergies. He did not feel that was to be considered at all. Avoidance of the offending foods is obviously the most realistic and optimum form of treatment. The problems occur when food is taken accidently, but it was up to us to provide as safe an environment as we possibly could. He said that Daniel was obviously thriving, and he put this down to the Nutramigen providing all the necessary nutrients. He felt that we were very fortunate that he enjoyed drinking it, as it really is difficult to persuade a toddler who has not been given Nutramigen from infancy to drink it, because it is so unpalatable. He made an appointment to see us in Out-Patients in one month's time, and would then be able to give me the results of most of the tests that had been done.

It was lovely to return home, to see Jeremy again. Robert had been visting us regularly in hospital keeping us informed of all the activities at home. Jeremy had been very happy with his grandparents, who had stayed in our home for one week, and then taken him back to their home in Somerset. He was settled and apparently unconcerned about his change of environment, or the whereabouts of the rest of us. At seven months he had not yet become very clingy and unsettled in other people's company, so it had been an appropriate time for me to leave him.

A couple of weeks later Daniel had an invitation to a little friend's birthday tea. He was excited and full of anticipation, although reluctant to leave my side when we got there. I had taken his tea for him: a sandwich, some plain crisps and a cake that I had baked, which was of course milk and egg-free. The dietitian at the hospital had given me a leaflet with about half a dozen cake and biscuit recipes, and it was one of these that I used. The other children were also eating jelly and ice cream. Daniel desperately wanted jelly, so I relented, thinking that one indiscretion was acceptable, even if we did have to suffer the consequences: probably a bad night. He thoroughly enjoyed it, and as he went home with his balloon and party hat he was excited and full of fun. That night he was very restless, and about 4 a.m. woke up anxious and having difficulty in breathing. In retrospect I can see that he was having his first asthmatic attack. It lasted for about three hours, and I found the easiest way to comfort him and help his breathing was to cuddle him upright in an armchair. He dozed and coughed and wheezed but it eventually wore off. I feel sure that the jelly was the culprit, as it was orange and contained the artificial colouring "Tartrazine", which is E102. I have since learned that one of the side effects of that particular colourant is wheezing. It seemed a sad price to pay for what was, on the face of it, such an innocuous party food.

We returned to out-patients in April and spent a long time discussing all the tests results, management, prognosis for the future etc. It appeared that Daniel's level of IgE (Immunoglobulin E) was very high. IgE is an antibody. The body manufactures antibodies as part of its normal defence mechanism. Many different types of antibodies are made, each designed to combat a specific foreign substance which enters the body and help it to return to a state of good health. If the invader is an allergen: i.e. a substance which has no effect at all in a non-allergic person, thus being quite harmless: in the allergic individual the antibody which is produced is called IgE. Each antibody is specific: that means that it will only react against the single allergen that it was produced to counteract. So, an IgE antibody against milk protein will react against proteins from any milk product, but not against egg or pollen protein. This is a very simplified explanation of IgE, but anyone who has an allergic child will surely have heard this term bandied about, and may be utterly confused by it.

Daniel's test results had been graded from 0 to 4, where 4 was the highest recording possible. Milk and egg white both produced a reaction of 4, and cats a reaction of 2.

The doctor plotted Daniel's height and weight on a graph and showed me that he was on the 90th percentile for both height and weight: in other words he was well above average in his growth, so his limited diet had had no adverse effect on his physical development. We discussed wearing a medic-alert disc, which in the event of an emergency situation could give the necessary information to a medical attendant. It was decided that this would be a good idea. Medic-alert forms are kept in G.P.s' surgeries. Part of the form is for completion by the parent, and a section needs to be completed by the family doctor. When asked about the future he reiterated that he really felt Daniel would improve before too long, but that allergy was a very new field of research, and that really the doctors were learning all the time from children like Daniel. It was difficult to forecast with any certainty, but he was hopeful. I was reassured by his obvious intent to answer all my questions honestly and as helpfully as possible. He was very thorough in a further examination of Daniel, and said he thought we should attend out-patients at three-monthly intervals for a while.

About a month after this visit, I had a phone call from the Children's Hospital one afternoon, asking me to take Daniel in to out-patients the next morning. There was no explanation, and I was naturally rather concerned and apprehensive as to why we were being called back. The appointment was to see the original dermatologist. She told me that a further test result had come back showing that Daniel had an allergy to wheat, and that we should eliminate this from his diet. I was quite bemused and asked whatever we were going to give him. She said I would be able to obtain "gluten-free" products from the chemist, and that there was a good range available now. I was aware of this, but wondered how many of those foods would also be milk, egg and additive-free.

The next day I rang our local hospital dietitian to ask her advice, and also went into the local chemist to look at their range of foods. Wheat is used so often, we take it for granted. It is in staple foods such as bread, cereals, biscuits etc.: certainly Daniel's staple foods: and I was at a loss to know how to replace them. We tried very hard for two weeks, but then asked for a further consultation. We saw the doctor on the Gastroenterology team who was now looking after Daniel, and he explained that in fact Daniel's wheat allergy test results had come back as a Grade 1, and that as he was not having any obvious reactions to it, it was more of a bother to remove it from his diet than to keep it in at the moment. He said that should the allergic response increase we would be aware of the same symptoms as occurred with milk and egg: i.e., urticaria, swelling, wheezing, etc. I felt very relieved at this advice as we had more than enough problems to be coping with.

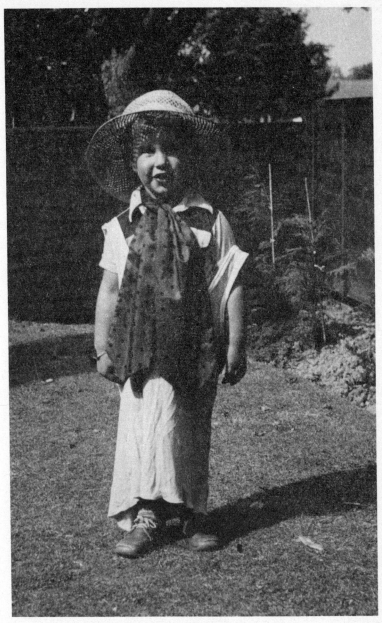

Anything for attention!

CHAPTER FIVE

At My Wit's End

The summer months brought a round of continuous infections for both boys. Jeremy seemed to be reacting to pollens, even though he wasn't yet one year old. He had the classic signs: puffy, swollen eyelids, runny nose, sneezing and wheezing. He had acute bronchitis several times, always accompanied by high fevers and difficulty in breathing. Both boys were prone to middle ear infections too. Jeremy was becoming very unsettled at night. He was noisy, demanding attention, restless and often appeared to be having colicky abdominal pain. Our nights were very broken once again, either through Jeremy's behaviour, or else because the repeated infections increased their irritability, disturbed their sleep and made them unhappy. I found the only way to get a few hours sleep was to take Jeremy out of his cot and cuddle him in a bed in his room. I desperately searched through his diet to try and find a possible cause of his problems, but he was drinking Nutramigen (advised by our G.P. in order to reduce potential accidents with Daniel) and he was on an additive-free diet. He drank dilute apple juice rather than orange, because his stools were always very loose and I felt apple juice might be less of an irritant than orange. The constant broken nights and repeated serious infections in the children were really getting me down again. I felt weary and depressed.

In December I took Jeremy to the doctor, because he had been passing a lot of mucus in his stools for weeks. His buttocks were often ulcerated. He had had several courses of oral and cream antibiotics to try to clear up nasty infected rashes on his bottom, and one day I was alarmed to see fresh blood streaked in his nappy. It was this that prompted me to return to the surgery. My G.P. felt that it was time for Jeremy to be referred to Birmingham too.

I spent Christmas in bed! My general health was obviously not at its best and I had an attack of flu and felt very sorry for myself. My parents, who had been invited for the festivities, ended up by being chief cooks and bottle washers. Jeremy was very unhappy and cried a great deal. He kept trying to crawl into bed with me. I can remember wondering whether apple juice could possibly be causing all his diarrhoea problems, and suggested that we tried him with pineapple juice as an alternative. Within three or fours days he was obviously improving. His bottom looked clearer than it had for weeks. He was sleeping better, and was a much happier little fellow.

The winter of 1981–82 was just about our lowest point. It was very cold and snowy. The snow lay on the ground for weeks, and I found it almost impossible to get the double buggy along the footpaths: consequently I didn't take the children very far at all. They had one chest or ear infection after another, and for weeks and weeks I didn't have a day when either one or both weren't having medicine.

One day I had a phone call offering me the opportunity of doing some part-time evening work. Part of me could not even conceive of it as I felt so weary and exhausted by the end of the day, but the other part of me was craving for some mental stimulation: something that was more than sick children and the same four walls. I accepted it. I really felt that my life was in need of an injection of something to boost me up. It was hard work to get organised enough to be out of the house by 6 p.m., but Robert was very supportive and helpful and could see how much I needed this alternative. It only worked out to be about one evening a week, and many times I went utterly exhausted, but returned refreshed, though obviously tired. Those evenings really helped to restore some balance to my life and I looked forward to them eagerly. Once again I was using some of my nursing skills and began to feel a useful member of society. I met a new circle of friends and began to feel I was getting out of the vicious circle I was trapped in. The whole family benefited as I was more able to cope with the problems at home having spent a few hours in an entirely different atmosphere. I am sure it is vitally important to become involved in some outside activity, however little time and commitment you can give, and however tired and unsociable you feel. In retrospect it is easy to recognise this, although at the time I must admit I found it extremely difficult to see the wood for trees.

I challenged Jeremy by reintroducing some apple juice one day, and he got frightening abdominal colic. His stools once again became profuse and offensive and he was unhappy. Apple juice certainly seemed to be the culprit.

At the end of January I was getting near the end of my tether. Jeremy was coughing and wheezing badly. I took him along to the surgery where the doctor listened to his chest very carefully but pronounced it clear. He felt his coughing was all due to nasal congestion and prescribed a decongestant. However, he had an ear infection, so he also gave me a prescription for antibiotics to clear that.

My parents were abroad on holiday, and all the bitterly cold weather had played havoc with their plumbing leading to many bursts which caused a great deal of damage in their house. Robert had been there at the weekend trying to help neighbours sort it out as best they could, and I had agreed to go down on the Tuesday in order to be there when they arrived home the following day, to light fires and explain what had happened. The house looked like a disaster area.

The journey down in the car was a nightmare. Jeremy was still coughing badly and he cried almost hysterically all the way. I stopped the car after about an hour and took him out of his seat to soothe and cuddle him. He took about half an hour to calm down, and I eventually got him back into his seat and gave him a drink. The screaming started again. I was desperate to get to my parents house, so carried on. I tried singing to him, saying all his favourite rhymes, but nothing worked and by the time we arrived Daniel had joined in too. I felt a nervous wreck.

During the next forty-eight hours Jeremy's behaviour

went from bad to worse. He screamed, threw things around the rooms, refused to eat and wouldn't let me out of his sight. I was at a complete loss to know how to deal with him. He slept about two hours in total, coughing and crying hysterically. He was still having his decongestant and antibiotics and I was also giving him analgesia thinking that his ear infection was causing him a lot of pain. My parents were very anxious about him – and me. I could feel myself very near to tears, and also dangerously near to physically hurting Jeremy. I couldn't understand his needs, and at the same time was obviously not satisfying his demands. He would not be pacified. He was utterly exhausted and yet would not rest. I felt absolutely incapable of doing anything with him. Daniel was being very naughty: it was one of the few ways he could get my attention as Jeremy was demanding everything I had.

I travelled home on the Thursday as we had a family appointment with the dentist. By the Friday morning I had had enough, after yet another night of no sleep. I rang my Health Visitor in desperation. I was in tears, tired out and very worried about Jeremy. I could not cope any longer. She came round to the house immediately and listened to my story. We had a cup of tea and I tried to convince myself that everything had got way out of proportion just because I was so physically worn out. Jeremy clung to me all the time, crying and coughing and Daniel did anything he could to get her attention. My Health Visitor said that she felt Jeremy was rather poorly and I explained that he had been examined at the beginning of the week but that his chest was clear, although he had an ear infection and was on antibiotics for that. She said she would call in to see my doctor and ask her to call and would pop back herself later.

The doctor called later in the morning, and once again all I could do was cry. That in itself told its own story. She was patient and sympathetic. Jeremy was on the dining table throwing anything he could onto the floor; Daniel was on the window ledge banging the windows. She said very kindly, "It doesn't do any harm to smack them you know!" I said that was all I seemed to be doing to them lately.

Daniel

She listened to Jeremy's chest and said he had a severe chest infection. The other ear was now badly infected and the eardrum bulging: so he was obviously in acute pain. The decongestant had a stimulant in it: something he very definitely did not need. A combination of all these factors was what was making him so desperately unhappy and unable to sleep. She advised that he had no more medicines which contained ephydrine (the stimulant and left me with a prescription for more antibiotics. She said she would like to see us again in five days; she was happy to call if I didn't feel up to going to the surgery. She said that I *must* get away for two or three nights to get some sleep, and reassured me that if my parents could come up to help, there would be plenty of support at the surgery, if it was necessary.

My Health Visitor called in again at lunch time and brought a form to enrol Daniel at the local Nursery School. He would be three years old in May and she and the doctor had discussed it and decided that we would all benefit if he could be accepted for mornings. I was horrified at the idea, partly because he had always been such a clingy child, partly because of his food and drink problems, and also because I just did not feel he could cope with five mornings a week. However, she pointed out that the environment would be a very "safe" one for Daniel to learn about his limitations. The children at the Nursery did not drink milk, which so many at the playgroup did, and should any crisis arise, it was situated next door to the surgery. If Daniel went in the mornings then I should be able to cope with just Jeremy, even if I was still getting little sleep. In other words, it would lessen the strain considerably. I was not convinced, but as May was three months away, I signed the forms in the knowledge that I had plenty of time to reconsider it.

My Health Visitor also told me that the doctor had rung Robert up at work to tell him that she had seen me during the morning and that I was under considerable strain and must get away for a rest. She told him that she would also ring the Hospital to chase up the appointment for Jeremy, as she was very worried about the number of serious infections he was getting so frequently.

When Robert arrived home from work we decided to ring my parents to ask if they could possibly come up to look after the boys while I had a break. We then rang my cousin to ask if I could go to stay with them, explaining the circumstances and the events that had led up to this. They live in a village in Nottinghamshire, and as they have no children I thought they would be ideal to spend a few quiet days with. It would be restful, and I knew they would be understanding and sympathetic. They assured me I would be very welcome.

I had three nights away from home, and I thought a great deal about the boys. However, not having to attend to them and not getting up at night did give me the rest I needed. I went for long walks with Pat and their three Afghan hounds. We shopped at leisure and browsed through sewing pattern books; we talked and discussed our mutually favourite hobbies: sewing, patchwork and cooking. I was very grateful for the care and attention I was given, but couldn't help wondering how everyone was getting on at home. They had not really missed me.

A week later Daniel was admitted to our local hospital. He had had a vomiting bug and had vomited copiously for about thirty-six hours. I had tried to give him glucose in water but whatever he took he could not tolerate. He began to look dehydrated. He had big black rings under his eyes and his skin was inelastic. He was cold and he looked very poorly. The doctor came out at 9 p.m. and said he felt he should be admitted. In hospital they tried to put up a drip four times: in both hands and both feet. Daniel struggled and fought, and the houseman was not very experienced. Daniel won every time, even though he was rather weak. They decided to leave him until morning when they would review him again. He was tolerating a few sips of water by then, and gradually through the day he managed more fluids. He was kept in hospital for just over two days, then I was allowed to take him home, for which I was very grateful. I was worried about his safety with food and drink, and felt much safer preparing and giving food myself.

A few days later we had an out-patients appointment in Birmingham for both boys, although primarily for Jeremy, as he had not been seen before. Robert came with us this time which was a great help, as both boys had to be undressed to be weighed and heighted. Trying to talk and listen whilst dealing with them was more than one could manage. Daniel was being a little unco-operative so the nurse tried to bribe him with a piece of chocolate! Luckily we prevented what would have been a very dangerous and distressing reaction.

They were both examined and we told our story once again, this time concentrating on Jeremy's problems. The doctor decided to admit both boys in order for Jeremy to have a full investigation and for Daniel's allergic state to be reassessed, and they were to be admitted the following week. I said I wished to stay in with them. The doctor said he felt I would be better going home to sleep where I would be able to have unbroken nights. However, I was very aware of how unhappy the boys would be if I wasn't available. It was also a forty-mile round trip for me to make between hospital and home, and I felt that that would have been just as tiring every day, so I was emphatic that I would like to stay with them.

It was an exhausting eight days. They were admitted to a medical ward where two cots were available, so that they could stay together. They had a series of intensive investigations and examinations. I also had a long chat with the medical social worker, but I did not find that she was terribly aware of the situation, even though she really did try to understand. When the houseman did his initial examination of them, I explained that they were both getting chest and ear infections very frequently, and fully expected one or both to be poorly within the next three or four days. Sure enough, Jeremy developed bronchitis with an ear infection, and Daniel started wheezing and had to be given nebulized Ventolin. They both started vomiting and between them ended up quite poorly, even though they were fit when admitted. They were eventually discharged as it was thought that Jeremy might be incubating measles with his chest infection and eyes which became rather puffy and sore. I quietly thought to myself, "This is what he does regularly at home, and is what I have been trying to tell everyone . . .", and of course he did not develop measles.

During the admission they both had their sinuses and chests X-rayed. In the X-ray department they were very apprehensive, and one radiologist cuddled Daniel while I held Jeremy on the table. Daniel had been crying and shouting but he suddenly became quiet. I heard the radiologist say, "And which colour would you like next?" and I saw her offering Daniel sweets: a mixture of Smarties and dolly mixtures. Thankfully he had eaten a dolly mixture the first time, and was just about to take a Smartie. I managed to stop him having it just in time. I had no wish to repeat the previous year's experience when he had been given the wrong food.

On the ward one day they decided to try Daniel with white fish as he had never eaten fish, and they felt it was the right place for his first challenge. The Staff Nurse flaked it onto his plate with his potatoes and said, "Doesn't it look dry: I'll just add a knob of butter", and with that she went to put some on his potato. Once again, I stopped her just in time. These two simple incidents illustrate how easy it is, without constant vigilance, to put Daniel in a potentially very hazardous situation. We, as parents, don't only have to think for ourselves, but for everyone else as well.

During this admission it was also suggested that I should be taught how to give an injection in the event of Daniel having a serious anaphylactic reaction at home, when a doctor might not be available instantly. I would be able to give a life-saving injection of adrenalin. I explained that I was a nurse, so I obviously knew how to give an injection. The boys were discharged with a variety of medicines for their current infections, and a supply of needles, syringes and adrenalin for emergency use only.

Daniel

Jeremy's allergy tests showed that he was "a very allergic child". He had high levels of IgE. His X-rays showed that he had chronic sinusitis, and he was obviously having problems as a result of repeated ear infections, so he was referred to an ear, nose and throat specialist. Daniel's "allergic state" had increased! What a pair! Even now I find it very hard to understand how we have managed to produce two boys with such acute allergies, when there is absolutely no family history of it.

It had occurred to me during this time that I might write a brief account of Daniel's allergy problems, and ask the Nursing Times whether they would be interested in publishing it. I had had two articles published by them in the past, so I knew that they liked my style of writing, and I felt the article would be of general interest. I wrote a two thousand word account and sent it off, wondering what the reaction would be. It was favourable, and they sent me the galley proofs to be checked quite quickly. The article was published a couple of months later.

I had recently read an article about the Attendance Allowance and wondered whether or not Daniel would be eligible for this, on supervisory grounds. I felt there was nothing to lose by applying for it, so duly collected the relevant form from the Department of Health and Social Security, filled it in and sent it off. We had a letter explaining that a doctor, who was not known to us, would be calling to examine Daniel and assess the situation. An appointment had been made. He spent one and a half hours with us, asking numerous questions about Daniel's problems and exactly how much attention and supervision were required for him. There were several pages of questions to be answered as well as a full statement of the exact nature of the problem, which had to be signed by me. The doctor was extremely thorough and methodical and although he was not allowed to give me any indication as to whether he felt we were entitled to the Attendance Allowance, I felt he had put forward as detailed a case as he possibly could. My thoughts were that if it wasn't granted, then we were obviously not entitled to it. He told me that it would be several weeks before we heard back from the Board who considered every application. It was about six weeks later when we heard that it had been granted. We were to receive the day-time allowance on the grounds that Daniel required constant supervision in order to prevent substantial danger to himself.

CHAPTER SIX

Coping With The Problems

It was a warm, sunny April day, and some friends were coming to tea. We had not seen them for nearly two years, so we were looking forward to hearing their news, and having a good chat. They had two children, older than Daniel and Jeremy, and the boys were eager to meet them. I spent the morning baking and preparing for tea. As usual when I was cooking I "batch-baked" and put the excess in the freezer, so when a friend called in during the morning, she looked around the kitchen and jokingly asked just how many were coming to tea. There always is a lot of preparation by the time I have baked cakes and biscuits, tarts, etc. for Daniel and then done the equivalent for Robert and any "normal" visitors. I use an egg white substitute to make meringues for Daniel and had cooked a batch of these and a batch of "ordinary" meringues. They were tea-spoon sized, and I had coloured Daniel's with pure blackcurrant juice so that they were easily identifiable from those made with egg white. I did not tell him I had made any, because I knew how much he enjoyed them and knew that it would be difficult to save them for tea. I also wanted to surprise him.

We thoroughly enjoyed the afternoon. The children played in the garden and were ready for tea when I called them in. They settled down with quite a lot of chatter and noise. With eight of us at the table including four young children there was a lot of activity. No one noticed Daniel get down from the table and go across to the hatchway where he had seen the cakes and meringues put carefully to one side. He helped himself to a meringue, unfortunately taking one of the wrong ones, and within seconds of biting into it he was coughing and spluttering. He had come back to the table and I could not understand what was wrong with him. Then I could see the remains of the meringue in his hand and I asked him if he had eaten it. He looked very frightened and nodded. His face and lips were swelling, and he started vomiting.

I asked Robert to ring the doctor, and carried Daniel into the bathroom. Robert got hold of the doctor on call. Luckily he was familiar with Daniel's problems and advised us to take him straight to casualty, and he would ring the casualty officer to say we were on our way.

We bundled Daniel into the car, and set off for the hospital. He was very swollen now, very anxious and wheezing badly. I realized that I hadn't given any explanation to our visitors and I had not said anything to Jeremy either. We had literally run out of the house leaving them all there, wondering what was happening.

In Casualty Daniel was given something to reduce the swelling, and a full history was taken. I explained that that was his very first ingestion of egg white. The tests he had had in Birmingham had shown that his allergic reaction to egg white was very severe, but I knew, quite emphatically, that he had never had egg in any form whatsoever, in any baby food or subsequent food. It was supposed that his sensitivity had come about again through my breast milk, as an infant. He vomited copiously and urticaria was evident around his neck, wrists and legs. His face and eyes were very swollen and his lips quite distorted. The casualty officer advised admitting him to the children's ward for observation, mainly to ensure that the allergic reaction did not become more severe and obstruct his breathing.

Robert returned home, to apologise for our dramatic disappearance and reassure everyone that Daniel was fine. The casualty officer looked in on Daniel during the evening. The swelling was beginning to subside, and there was apparently no further danger, so she was happy for him to be discharged. However, as a precaution, she gave me some hydrocortisone, needles and syringes in case of a delayed reaction, and told me not to hesitate to take him back if we were at all worried.

Daniel took it all in good part, but we both learnt from the situation: Daniel, that he must always ask before he eats anything, and I became very aware of how important it was to explain to him which was his food, particularly when there was the possibility of a similar situation occurring. Robert and I had perhaps also become rather complacent about Daniel and his problems, and this episode certainly served to remind us that we always had to be vigilant, particularly when there were visitors in the house and our attention could easily be diverted.

One other effect that this episode had was to illustrate to friends and neighbours just how serious Daniel's problems were. We were constantly saying "Please don't give him anything to eat or drink; no sweets, no biscuits; don't let him touch this or that; don't, don't, don't . . ." I am sure I was thought of as being a very fussy, faddy mother, and one effect of this regrettable accident was to show that he really would end up in hospital very quickly, if given the wrong food. They had seen it happen now, and Daniel's problems had gained credibility.

One day I had bought a packet of three new bath sponges from the chemist. We put them in the bath that night with the boys, and they bathed and played with their toys. When the water was let out of the bath and the boys dressed in their pyjamas, we noticed that the tide mark was slightly coloured where some of the dye had come out of the sponge. One part of the bath had a blue stain and another a pink one. Within a couple of hours of going to bed, Daniel woke up coughing and wheezing. His nose was completely blocked, the upper part of his face very swollen, his eyes puffy and almost closed. He was frightened and finding it very difficult to breathe. It seemed that he had reacted to the dye in the water. The reaction subsided very gradually over the next few hours, and when he eventually woke in the morning he was back to normal. This type of reaction has happened many times. Occasionally we can pin-point a probable culprit, but many times it is not at all obvious what has caused the reaction. All we can do is to reassure him, sit him up in a chair and read to him, or at least try to divert his attention from his obvious discomfort, and give him Ventolin for his wheezing.

Robert was very anxious that we should be able to protect Daniel from being offered food and drink which could produce severe reactions. He was only three years old and could not be expected to know what he could accept and what wouldn't be safe for. What a responsibility! So he decided to see if he could get some badges designed for Daniel to wear which would give a visual reminder that people must not offer him food, drinks, sweets etc., due to food allergies. The following three slogans were chosen: "I am violently allergic to many foods", "No foods, drinks or sweets please. Severe food allergies" and "Serious food allergies. Please *do not* feed me". These were mounted onto brightly coloured card and made into badges, using a badge press. Whenever Daniel goes anywhere where he is not known, or where he may get lost, or where there is any chance that strangers might offer him food, he wears a couple of badges. By wearing two, slightly differently worded, I feel that it probably adds emphasis to the problem, rather than appearing to be just a gimmick.

Daniel was still having frequent bouts of diarrhoea, almost always preceded by tummy ache. Every day he would complain of pain and although it did not incapacitate him unduly, it was obviously causing a fair amount of discomfort. The diarrhoea occurred two or three times a day, and probably three or four days a week. However he continued to thrive, obviously gaining adequate nutrition from his diet, plus Nutramigen.

With Daniel's diet being so limited, it was, and still is, virtually impossible to buy much in the way of commercially prepared foods for him, either because of the artificial additives, or else because so many foods contain egg or milk in one form or another. This meant that I had to think up new ideas and adapt recipes, particularly for snacks and treats and puddings. Sometimes my experiments were well received, and sometimes virtually totally

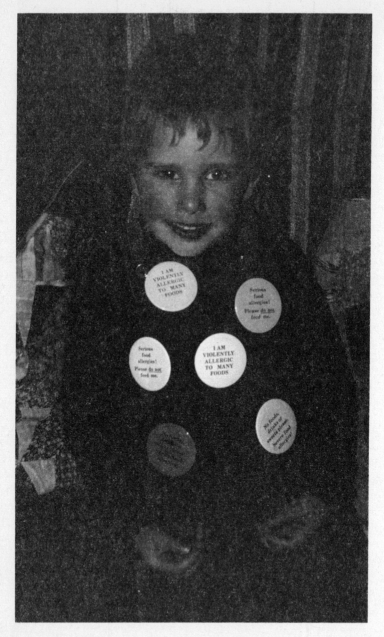

Please do not feed this child

ignored. You can rely upon a child to be quite honest in his judgement: a good indication that it has been accepted is a request for seconds. When I saw "milk free" recipes advertised anywhere I used to send off for them, but was invariably disappointed, as in most cases a milk substitute such as goat's milk or soya milk, was used as a replacement. I found I could not use Nutramigen in the same way, because of its very strong flavour, and also because Daniel just would not accept its use in cooking, the recipes were often of no use to me.

During the month of May Daniel was to attend the Nursery for a couple of hours each Wednesday morning. This was to give a gentle introduction and allow him to become familiar with the environment and routine. On our first morning his attention was caught by the large painting easel and paints. A nursery helper showed him where the plastic aprons were kept, so that he could put one on to protect his clothes, and he had a very enjoyable time covering a big piece of paper with bright colours. He was shown around all the other activities and listened to the morning story. He was anxious that I was always in sight, but ran eagerly from one activity to another. The following week he had tonsillitis, so missed that session, but he went the next Wednesday morning and again appeared to settle fairly well. When he started each morning I stayed for a few minutes, getting him involved in particular activity, but he was always extremely upset when I left him. This happened for several weeks and it was quite distressing for both of us, but suddenly he decided to accept it and for the eighteen months he spent there he played and "worked" hard. He was a solitary child: happy in his surroundings, sociable with staff and children, but far preferring his own company to that of the crowd. I was most impressed by the kindness and attention given to the children. The staff were extremely careful that Daniel should not eat, drink or touch anything that might harm him. He had his own tin of biscuits which he used to have on the odd occasions that the other children had a treat: for instance birthdays, and special occasions when cakes had been taken in. The staff were always impressed by his accepting attitude. He never appeared to mind the fact that he could not eat the treats the other children were given. Each morning he took his own drink of juice, while the other children drank orange squash.

At an out-patient appointment during the summer the doctor suggested that I tried the boys with plain chocolate: partly because it was a "treat", something that was quite rare in the food line, and partly as it was a good source of energy. Each lunch time when Daniel came home from Nursery, they each had one square of dark chocolate with their drink of Nutramigen. They loved it, and I was definitely out of favour if I had inadvertently run out. However, quite insidiously their behaviour began to deteriorate. They became very excitable and constantly noisy and more aggressive, and they argued incessantly. Our nights became very broken once again. Jeremy, particularly, was getting more frequent asthmatic attacks, and the amount of antibiotics required for ear and chest infections was really quite worrying. Both boys had developed sensitivities to several antibiotics. Daniel had had extensive urticaria with his last course of penicillin. When the urticaria had subsided it had left him with his skin covered in tiny blisters, which irritated him, and lasted for about a week. They had both reacted to erythromycin, erupting in nasty, infected spots, and Daniel had also been incontinent of urine day and night for the whole of his last course of erythromycin. Jeremy's skin took a long time to clear up, and in fact he developed impetigo on his face before the rash finally disappeared. Jeremy also erupted in a rash with Septrin on the last occasion that that had been given, and Daniel has subsequently reacted by having asthma with Septrin. His wheezing increased throughout the course, becoming quite alarming and not responding to his normal treatment, but within twenty-four hours of completing the Septrin, his asthma stopped.

Once again Robert and I looked to the boys' diet,

wondering if there was some item which could be causing the disruptive nights, and possibly the frequent infections too. Chocolate was the obvious culprit, so we removed it, and the effect of that was quite dramatic. Nights became calmer and we all started sleeping again, and the boys' general health very definitely improved.

At an out-patients appointment later in the year, the doctor looked at Daniel and Jeremy who were playing quietly on the floor in the consulting room. "What have you done to them?" he asked. "I usually go home with a migraine when you have been to the clinic!"

I knew exactly what he meant, as I dreaded the hospital visits myself. I explained about the chocolate and what a vast improvement we had had, gradually cutting out additives, salicylates, and now stopping the chocolate too. Everything had seemed to get a lot worse, even with the tiny amount of chocolate they had been having, but the consequence of its removal was there to be seen. I was very pleased that he had commented on it quite spontaneously, before I had had a chance to mention it. He explained that in chocolate there was substance very similar to adrenalin, in minute quantities, and the boys' sensitivities were such that even the tiniest amount was obviously sufficient to aggravate their nervous system. As always he examined them thoroughly, and took all the details of the various happenings since he had last seen us. Chocolate was definitely not to be reintroduced for at least one year, and he said he would review it then.

CHAPTER SEVEN

"What Can I Give Him Today?"

When we first lived in Yorkshire we made friends with two
Canadians, Brian and Joanna, who were over in England
for one year's study at York University. We had maintained our friendship over the years, and had spent a
glorious summer holiday in Canada with them in 1978, the
year before Daniel was born. They were now back in
England for a further year and had two children
themselves. In October they came to stay with us for a few
days, and it was one day while we chatted about the
problems of finding new ideas for varying Daniel's diet
that the idea of producing a recipe booklet began to grow.
Brian had his own computer and word processor, and he
offered to do the print-out for me, if I managed to get one
under way.

I had already collected many recipes which I used
regularly and the thought of planning all these together
into a booklet was quite exciting. I was not sure how to go
about getting it printed, or how to advertise it, but those
were problems I could cope with as they arose. I decided to
limit the book to 50 recipes, all of which would be milk, egg
and additive free. I had no intention of producing menus,
or of providing ideas for a "balanced diet", but rather to
concentrate on cakes, biscuits, puddings and snacks. We
decided to include a badge kit at the back of the book so
that parents could make up their own brightly coloured
badges if they wanted. The title "What Can I Give Him
Today?" presented itself quite naturally. I said it, in
desperation, most days of the week!

Brian and Jo worked very hard and produced the layout
for me during a weekend of intensive work. I had obtained
a couple of quotes from printers, and we decided to have

500 printed initially, not knowing really what the demand would be. I wrote about twenty letters to various allergy societies, journals and publications which I felt would reach the population who might benefit from the booklet. With each letter I sent a copy, so that it could be examined and reviewed. The project was not intended to be a profit making venture at all, but rather a self-help idea. Knowing for myself just how difficult it was to get hold of milk and egg-free recipes, I felt the need must be there for countless other families too. We worked out our expenses, because although I did not particularly want to make a profit, neither did I want to run at a loss. We added on the price of package and postage and a donation for the H.A.C.S.G. and found that we could realistically price the booklet at 85p. This I felt was within the means of most people who might request it.

I was very excited the day they arrived, and also slightly anxious that we might be left with 500 recipe booklets which nobody else wanted! I took one along to the baby clinic to show to my Health Visitor, and she asked if I had told the local newspaper about it. I said that I hadn't, and she immediately rang the office and explained about it. Her husband was a photographer for the paper, so she knew the staff. Within a couple of days a journalist came round, and I told her our story. She took some photos of Daniel and I cooking in the kitchen and tasted some "Daniel" biscuits. The article was printed in our local Weekly News that week, and that was the start of a very busy month. Many days I had phone calls from newspapers asking if they could come and do an article. One afternoon the telephone rang, and it was one of the producers of BBC Breakfast Time Television. They had heard about the recipe booklet and wanted to know whether they could do a feature. I was speechless. I really had no idea that all this publicity might arise, so quickly, from a local press article.

A couple of days later Central Television rang at 9 o'clock in the morning. They had seen an article in a national newspaper, and were keen to follow it up. They came the same day and did an interview, as well as filming the baking in the kitchen and Daniel playing out in the garden. The crew consisted of the programme presenter, a lighting man, a camera man and a sound recordist. They were a friendly, happy crew who did their best to put me at my ease, but I really didn't have time to be nervous. When Robert arrived home from work that evening he was sorry that he had missed all the activity.

In the next few days, following the Central Television News programme, I received about two hundred letters in the post. Many of these letters contained detailed accounts of families coping with allergy problems, often unsupported by medical help, and struggling to find out as much information as possible. Answering letters and sending off booklets was quite demanding on my time, but I thoroughly enjoyed it. Most days the boys raced to the door when they heard the letters plopping through the letter box and I was met with cries of, "There are hundreds today, Mummy!" They got as much pleasure out of opening them as I did. It is now two years since I first advertised the booklet, and I have sold two thousand from home. The need is evident, and I am only too pleased to have been able to help some people in some small measure.

A day or two after the television programme we had an out-patient appointment in Birmingham. I was slightly anxious about the reaction of the doctors at the hospital, because we had received a great deal of help and understanding from them and I didn't want to antagonise them or jeopardise our relationship in any way. I did not want them to feel we had sensationalized Daniel's problems, because we hadn't. The Press and the Media seem to be law unto themselves, and any feature that they do can end up rather distorted, bearing little resemblance to the initial problem. However, to be fair, Central Television produced an accurate account of Daniel's allergies, cutting very little of what I told them. The dietitian was the first person I met in the large out-patients hall.

"I saw you on the television on Wednesday night," she

said. "It was very good. Can I have a copy of the recipe booklet?". She was most interested, particularly in the "additive-free" angle of the recipes, as she said they had recently started many of their eczema patients on additive-free diets, and were having some good results.

When the doctor called us in, I took the bull by the horns and decided to ask him if he had seen the programme. He said he hadn't seen it, but his secretary had, and she had told him all about it. I asked him if he minded. "Not at all," he said, and continued that he felt "allergy" had rather a bad name at the moment particularly after all the press publicity on the "total allergy syndrome', which had been widely speculated on in the papers and on radio and television. He felt it was good for the public to see that allergy was a serious problem which could easily disrupt family life, and that it was necessary to see how people coped with it, and were leading normal lives in spite of all their problems. I was reassured by his attitude as I would have been extremely upset if he had taken offence. He asked me for a couple of books, as he felt he would be able to recommend it to other patients.

About a week later the BBC film crew arrived, and once again I was interviewed and demonstrated some more cooking. Daniel was getting quite used to being photographed, and took it all very much in his stride. I don't think he had any idea of what it was all about. We just explained to him that because he had a very funny tummy and wasn't able to eat many foods that other boys and girls could eat he was really rather special, and other people were interested to hear about him and see what kind of recipes his Mummy cooked for him.

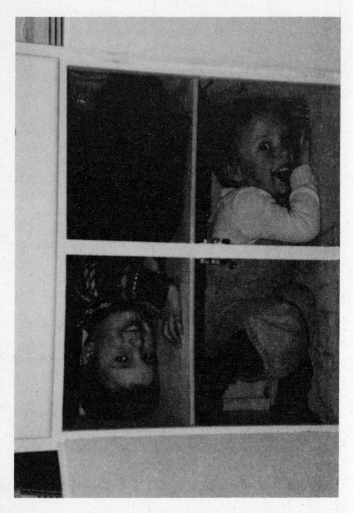

Kitchen devils

CHAPTER EIGHT

Hidden Ingredients

Daniel's fourth birthday was at the end of May. I took him to Nursery and then took Jeremy on to the surgery, as he was not at all well. He had a high temperature and was coughing badly. The doctor said he had a chest infection, so on our way home I called in at the chemist to collect his antibiotics. The health food shop was close by, and I popped in quickly just to see if there were any "treats" I could buy for Daniel's birthday. I picked up a Carob Crunch bar and read the ingredients on the wrapper. There didn't appear to be anything in the list that Daniel could not have, so I bought two and took them home. That would be a nice surprise for him. I was always excited if I thought I had found something new that he could have. Just to see the pleasure written all over his face was reward enough.

When Daniel and I got home he bounced inside, happy and chattering. I showed him the Carob Crunch bar and he asked if he could try it. Cautiously he bit a tiny piece of the corner, as he always did when trying anything new. I thanked Hazel, the neighbour who had come in to look after Jeremy whilst I collected Daniel, and as she walked down the path, Daniel cried out that his mouth hurt. I thought he must have bitten his tongue or cheek. Then he cried that his throat was hurting. He had swallowed what he had in his mouth. I became alarmed as he started coughing and retching. Within half a minute his face had swollen and his eyes almost closed. His lips were oedematous and he was vomiting. I read the ingredients on the label again. There was definitely no milk or egg listed, and yet his reaction belied that fact. I rang Hazel just so that she could see the transformation from a happy, boisterous child, to this miserable swollen little boy.

63

Daniel was frightened and unhappy. He was wheezing badly and sat pathetically on the settee.

The swelling subsided over the next few hours, but the wheezing continued for several days. I decided to write to the manufacturers of the Carob Crunch to ask them to detail very specifically every single ingredient in it. I explained about Daniel's problems, and said that naturally I was concerned in case he was reacting to some new item of food. It took them seven weeks to reply to me, but there in the list was "skimmed milk". The carob coating around the bar contained the milk, but this had not been listed on the packaging. I rang the Weights and Measures Department locally to ask their advice, and to see whether in fact the manufacturers were breaking the law by not listing every ingredient. I was informed that if an ingredient is part of a compound ingredient, such as the carob coating, then if it is less than 25% of that compound, by law it does not have to be listed. Well, if that was the law, I had to accept it, but judging by the tiny amount Daniel had eaten, and the allergic response he had had, I questioned whether or not the milk was less than 25%. The gentleman I spoke to was extremely helpful and sympathetic and said he would ask their laboratories to analyse the content for me. I was grateful, as we rely heavily on the accuracy of the listing of ingredients on foods. Had Daniel just launched in and eaten a big piece, I feel sure he could have been in serious trouble.

Months later I learnt that the analysis showed the milk content to be greater than 25% and that the Weights and Measures Department would be informing the manufacturers of this point. At a later date I received a letter from the County Trading Standards Department explaining the course of action they had taken. I felt very satisfied that the matter has been dealt with in a thorough and understanding way. The letter stated:

In view of the analyst's report on this product I contacted the company responsible for the packaging and labelling of this product and informed them that in our opinion the labelling did not comply with the Regulations and advised them on the correct labelling. I also passed on all the information to the Trading Standards Department in Surrey where the company is situated. This is our usual practice in cases such as this, as it is easier and more effective for the local department to visit the premises of the company and fully advise them in relation to the ingredients, and the methods used to make the product. It is also easier for the local department to ensure that the advice is being followed and that the labelling is corrected as soon as possible. There is an inevitable delay in the introduction of amended labelling due to the printing of new packaging material, and stocks of the product held at wholesale and retail level, which is in the old packaging. I did, however, stress to both the company and the local Trading Standards Department that this was not, as it might first appear, a labelling technicality, but could have very serious consequences for anyone such as your son who ate products containing milk products which are not declared.

Daniel's tummy aches and diarrhoea had increased. He seemed to be complaining after almost every meal, and often had to rush off to the toilet straight after eating. We got used to him shouting out, "squits again Mummy!" but it was rather disconcerting if we had visitors in the house. I had started a food diary again, really to see if I could pin-point any possible causes, but as it was happening so frequently it just was not possible. He wasn't ill, and showed no signs of weight loss or apathy at all. It was just a nuisance: and obviously not very pleasant for Daniel. We could see urticarial weals on him often, but usually were unable to find the cause. He regularly had swollen lips or a swollen eye, when he had obviously touched some item he was sensitive to. I had to be very careful when I was baking not to touch him before washing hands. One hot summer day, when he just had little shorts on, I had been grating some cheese when I heard him screaming outside. I ran out and picked him up: he had fallen off his trike. Unfortunately, he then not only had grazed knees and elbows to contend with, but also itchy urticaria on his trunk, from where I had been handling the cheese. We have to be scrupulous about washing down the kitchen surfaces and tables, as, like any other child, Daniel is constantly touching, leaning against and swinging from them. One day the milk man dropped a pint of milk outside the door. The bottle smashed, and the milk splashed everywhere. Of all the houses in the street, it had to be ours!

The boys had always asked us for a drink of "milk" if they wanted Nutramigen, and both Robert and I had several times gone to the fridge, and even got as far as pouring out a drink of milk, before realizing our mistake. So we encouraged them to ask us for Nutramigen, just to emphasize that it was Nutramigen and not milk that we were supposed to be giving them. Hopefully that would help to minimize those potentially disastrous occasions that always left me shaking like a leaf.

Daniel had several invitations to friends' parties. He used to wear a couple of badges warning people not to give him food; but he was never happy to stay on his own, often displaying anxiety about his food being all right. I prepared all his food and took it along to the host with precise instructions on what he could and could not do. Invariably, I ended up staying to help supervise, so that Daniel felt more relaxed and able to enjoy himself. At one particular party all the children were given ice cream in a cone after their tea, and they went charging round the garden chasing each other with their ice creams. I was horrified. If anyone bumped into Daniel and he got ice cream on his face, the reaction could be catastrophic. Under any other circumstance this would have been harmless, enjoyable fun, but I watched like a cat on hot bricks. Daniel thankfully kept well away, and played quietly on a swing.

At our next out-patients appointment the doctor decided to start Daniel on Nalcrom. This had been discussed at previous visits, but it was felt that while we could monitor his diet and activities so closely, we could, as far as possible, protect him from being given unsafe foods. Nalcrom is oral Intal, a drug manufactured by Fisons, and given to help prevent allergic reactions in the gut, just as inhaled Intal helps to prevent allergic reactions in the lungs, i.e. asthma. It has to be taken regularly before every meal. If a dose is forgotten, then the previous dose does not offer continued protection, so regular intake is essential. The doctor felt that with all the abdominal pain and recurrent diarrhoea that Daniel was perhaps reacting, less severely, to many other foods. The Nalcrom could then help to reduce the symptoms. He would also be starting school in a few months time, and it was felt that the Nalcrom could help to protect him from a serious reaction should he be tempted to, or even accidentally, eat some "wrong food". It comes in capsule form and Daniel accepted them readily, swallowing them with no fuss at all. During the next four weeks his diarrhoea increased, and I became quite anxious about him. Thinking about it carefully, I realized that it was since he had started the Nalcrom that he was getting much more diarrhoea. Our G.P. sent a stool specimen off to the Path. Lab. just as a precaution, but the result was negative. So I rang the hospital to speak to our doctor there. He was at a case conference and was not available, so I explained to his secretary exactly what was happening and she assured me that he would ring the following morning. When he rang back he had already been in contact with Fisons, to see whether this could be a side effect of the drug. Apparently they had had one or two cases, particularly in young children, reacting like this. They advised stopping it completely until the diarrhoea ceased, then recommencing with just one capsule per day for a week, gradually increasing to four a day over the next month. By the time he was having two a day the diarrhoea had started again, but we persisted and after about six weeks his gut seemed to settle down and accept the Nalcrom.

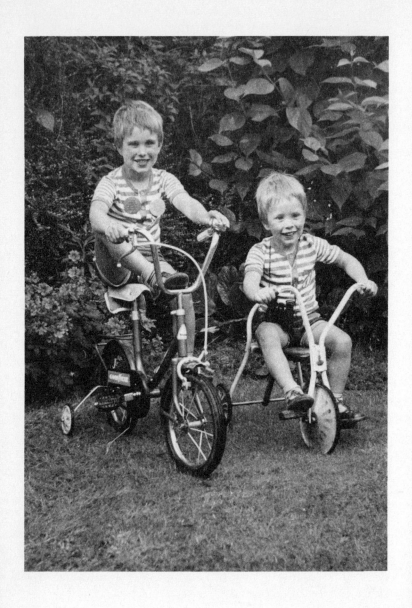

Always on the go

CHAPTER NINE

Another House Move

Robert had gained promotion in his job. He had been Head of Physics in his school, and had gained promotion to Head of the Science Department in a Comprehensive School in Cheltenham, so we knew that once again we would be moving house, to Gloucestershire. The whole process of house hunting and physically moving house was much more of a hassle that it had been three years earlier. Robert's new job started in September, and we did not actually move house until December, so those few months were rather hard for all of us. The boys missed their Daddy, and were overjoyed to see him at weekends. They had frequent chest infections, and several asthmatic attacks, and without a car to take them to the surgery I had to rely on neighbours helping me out. Everybody was extremely helpful, and I was even able to continue my evenings at work due to the kindness of one of our close neighbours, being more than willing to babysit for me.

I was excited about the move, but also rather apprehensive about all the changes that would have to take place. Our present G.P.s knew us very well, and were aware of all the problems. They had been extremely supportive throughout our three years there. Would a new G.P. practice be so understanding and supportive? We would have to start again explaining Daniel's problems to all new acquaintances, neighbours etc. Would they just think that we were terribly fussy and overprotective? Daniel would be starting a new school where nobody knew him. Would they be sensitive to his circumstances? Would he be allowed to take a packed lunch? Would we have to change hospital consultants, or could we still travel up to Birmingham? They knew us so well, and the thought of starting all over again with a new set of paediatricians was a daunting thought. However these were all bridges that we would have to cross as we arrived at them.

We were sorry to be leaving Warwickshire. We had made some very good friends, and had been very settled and happy there. We had lived through some of the most harrowing months of our lives, but had always found sympathy and understanding. I was particularly sorry to be leaving my job. In retrospect I could see very clearly how much I had depended on those early evenings, which offered me a respite from the strain of the problems at home. I had made some very good friends, and thoroughly enjoyed the work, which had given me back an element of independence, as well as an outlet for my emotions. However, we were making progress. The boys' allergy problems seemed to be well under control, and we were in a more stable family situation making the move this time.

We moved house in December, two weeks before Christmas, and worked very hard during that fortnight to get the house organised for the Christmas festivities. My G.P. had given me a letter to give to the new doctor we would be registering with, just giving a brief introduction to Daniel, prior to his notes being transferred. I needed to be able to get regular prescriptions for his Nutramigen and Nalcrom, and it was also important that he should be aware that a serious allergic reaction could occur, requiring immediate attention.

We had already been in touch with the school we had chosen for Daniel to attend, and I took him up to meet the Head Teacher and his class teacher. They had already received a letter from our old G.P. giving very explicit details of his problems, and could not have been more helpful or understanding. They asked many questions about what it was safe for Daniel to do in the classroom: particularly at milk time, cookery lessons, lunch times, etc. The Headmistress was happy to give Daniel his Nalcrom capsule prior to him having his lunch, and it was decided that it would be safer for him to be out of the classroom altogether when the other children had their milk, so at these times he goes across to the secretary's office and reads or draws for ten minutes.

One day his class teacher asked if I could take in some ingredients that Daniel could use in a cookery lesson. She said he was always very patient, and never complained, but of course he didn't have anything to do with the cooking because of the margarine and/or eggs used. The children always shared the results of the cookery lesson too, which of course Daniel could not do. So now and again they bake a "Daniel recipe", using his milk-free margarine and other ingredients, and which all the children then enjoy afterwards. Daniel confided one day, "I was allowed to have two buns today because they were my special ones!"

Adjusting to school life has been a major hurdle for Daniel, as it obviously is for many children. He is, by nature, a rather insecure child: he needs to be very familiar with routine, people and situations in order to feel confident and be able to participate. He is quite suspicious of anything new and emotionally rather immature. He easily bursts into tears, and often appears unsure of himself. However, in many other ways he is mature for his age and takes things seriously, with a great deal of responsibility. He has settled down well, and although he doesn't appear to have any special friends, he does seem to mix well generally, and is enthusiastic about his lessons, as well as play times.

In January we went back to the Children's Hospital in Birmingham. As always we discussed all aspects of the boys' health and I registered concern at the amount of wheezing Daniel was having. Oral Ventolin took a long time to work and we had tried an inhaler, used through a polystyrene coffee cup held up to his face. When he was very distressed he would not tolerate this, so we had no method of giving him instant relief. It was decided to try him with a Bricanyl Nebuhaler. This proved to be very successful, and Daniel is happy to use his "space breather" as he calls it. The amount of wheezing he has had in the six months since we have moved has increased, but it is easily controlled using the Nebuhaler, and as yet has not required further medical intervention. I don't feel that the wheezing is as a result of environmental changes, either in locality or our house, but rather just Daniel's physical state. The amount of tummy aches, often associated with diarrhoea has started to increase again. Whether this is an indication that his tolerance of certain foods is lowering and/or the Nalcrom is not working for him so well, is pure speculation. Physically he looks extremely healthy, and he enjoys life to the full. He walks just over a mile each way to school most days, coping perfectly adequately with only the usual moaning and groaning any five year old would do. Mentally as well as physically he is maturing.

I remember a discussion I had with the doctor in Birmingham one day, when he said that there might be a time when Daniel might decide to "experiment" with food: this could well prove a very serious situation. I had been saying that I was surprised at how well he accepted his very limited diet. He never seemed to bother that other children round him, particularly at parties, on outings etc., were eating ice cream, chocolate biscuits, brightly coloured cakes, sweets, etc. His remarks have always been at the back of my mind, and several times recently Daniel has wistfully said, "I wish I could try some yoghurt", or "It would be nice to have a piece of cheese". We commiserate with him, and explain that he has a very "funny tummy" and really is rather special. We also stress the serious reactions he has had and highlight the worse effects, just hoping this may serve as a deterrent. I feel that at the moment he is too frightened to consider "trying" one of the forbidden foods, but that as he gets older he may be pressurized into it by his peers. Children can be incredibly unkind to each other, and if he was taunted and teased into such a situation, then who knows what the outcome might be.

Hay fever, as yet, has not been one of Daniel's problems, although he is obviously a prime candidate in the future. This year, at the beginning of the pollen season in May, he came indoors at tea-time, sneezing, with a blocked nose and conjunctivitis. One eye was extremely swollen, and during the next couple of hours practically closed. He was terribly distressed by the soreness and grittiness of his eyes, which he could not stop rubbing, and also by the pain in his soft palate. He had great difficulty breathing through his nose. These symptoms persisted for forty-eight hours, and then gradually subsided, and as yet have not returned this hay fever season. So, quite what the irritant was is not at all obvious, as the pollen counts have been high, but apart from occasional wheezing and the usual blocked nose there have been no other symptoms.

As a result of our last visit to the Children's Hospital, Daniel's Nalcrom has been increased to two capsules before meals, and Jeremy has been started on Nalcrom, just one capsule before meals. This is in response to increasing attacks of abdominal pain and diarrhoea.

Daniel is now six years old. He has learnt to live with his problems very well indeed, and leads as normal a life as any other child, with very strict control over his diet, and constant vigilance in the kitchen and where food is concerned. He is very aware of his problems, and on the whole accepts them very well. He has needed a great deal of medical attention in these six years, but is very trusting of his doctors, both general practitioners, and hospital staff. This I feel pays tribute to them and the way they have handled him. We have been very fortunate in our medical care, and this has gone a long way in helping us to understand his problems, and to cope with them sensibly.

Life always seems busy, if only from the catering point of view. I watch other mothers enviously as I shop. They go along the shelves, and into the freezers, stocking their trolleys with a variety of packet and convenience foods. That is not for us. I always have to think well in advance. When I run out of fish fingers I have to make a new batch. When Daniel's cake and biscuit tins are empty, I have to start baking. If we go out for the day, we can never pop into a cafe for a snack, we always have to pack up before we set off. If we go away to friends for weekends, I still have to make sure that we take enough "Daniel food" with us: that means such foods as bread, juice, cake, biscuits, Nutramigen, perhaps an "uncontaminated" honey pot (i.e. we cannot use one that may have had a buttery knife put into it). Daniel inevitably wheezes in a strange home, so I must make sure that we carry his Bricanyl Nebuhaler, plus their Nalcrom, Piriton, Ventolin – and somewhere in our luggage the emergency adrenalin kit!

Holidays always have to be self catering, and catering for Daniel for a fortnight in advance is no mean task. I take nearly all the boys' food, and Rob and I eat "convenience" foods to lessen the work load. On one occasion when we had stocked up at the local supermarket, I had asked the boys to carry a sliced loaf each. The ensuing conversation between them was quite delightful because they were amazed that the bread was already in slices in the packet. They had never seen this strange phenomenon before. It really would be very nice to have a holiday where we are totally looked after for a week or two, but the catering problems would be enormous, and at the moment this is just not for us. Like many other families for a variety of reasons, we must accept that "a change is as good as rest."

For the last four years, I have acted as a local contact for the Hyperactive Children's Support Group. In the first instance this meant having my name listed in the Journal and locally as being willing to be a "pair of ears" for other mothers who were having problems with their hyperactive children. I would be able to offer advice about diet and foods, on the "safe" foods to use and on helpful shops to buy from; also to offer continued support after children have commenced on additive-free diets. Having trained and worked as a Health Visitor I am very well aware that behaviour problems in children can occur for numerous reasons, whether they are social, physical, psychological, environmental or dietary. Obviously, problems which could result from any of these causes need proper diagnosis for optimum results. Having said that, the vast majority of people that have contacted me have usually done this as a last resort. They have often been through the gamut of the conventional approaches to modifying their children's anti-social behaviour, and sometimes sampled some of the unconventional methods too. They may have heard from friends, or read in the Press, that their children's diet could be the cause of their unruly, disruptive behaviour, and they are desperate for help.

To suggest to a family that they remove artificial additives from their diet is not posing any nutritional risk to the children. All one is doing is removing items from the diet which are not necessary and have no food value. In most cases there are perfectly acceptable alternatives. However, I am aware that it does put quite a strain on the family because planning meals and shopping initially becomes far more of a chore and a challenge. But, as they become familiar with "safe" foods and their knowledge of the listed ingredients on packaged items increases, so the problems are gradually overcome. The families are usually very well motivated and are willing to put up with the strain and inconvenience. In young children behaviour changes are usually quite dramatic, over a very short period of time, usually days. In older children, changes take much longer, often several weeks, and these families need lots of support and help.

For any family, following a total exclusion diet creates quite a lot of social problems, but if as a result of that diet they have a child who remains physically well, and behaviourally and emotionally well-balanced, then those efforts are surely well rewarded. If artificial additives have been the cause of the child's problems, then it is usually possible to demonstrate this very easily. Once they have been excluded from the diet, and behaviour and sleep patterns have all settled down, then to reintroduce them into the diet, even on one occasion only, is usually sufficient to demonstrate a return of all the old problems.

When we moved to Gloucestershire, I noticed that there were two other contacts for the Hyperactive Children's Support Group, near by: Heather and Florence. I got in touch with them, and it was interesting for us to share our experiences, and to offer support to each other. One day, the Social Services Department rang Heather offering her the use of a large room with play facilities and kitchen in a Family Centre, for one afternoon a week. This was done with a view to organising a play/advice session for families with pre-school hyperactive children. She rang me, very excited, and asked what I thought about it. It really seemed far too good an offer to turn down.

Obviously a lot of commitment goes into a project such as this, and Heather and Florence, and subsequently many other members, have given a great deal of time and energy towards this venture. We have had fund raising coffee mornings, initially to buy a library of books which could be lent out, and also to provide a Christmas party for the pre-school children who came regularly to the Group. Its aims were to offer information, advice and support to mothers coming, with hyperactive and allergic children, and also to provide a "play group" for these children. So often they are not accepted into normal toddler/playgroups because of their disruptive behaviour. Some weeks are very quiet, others are extremely busy and noisy. We find that some mothers attend regularly, and obviously find this very supportive. Others come just once and have a long chat and go away with lots literature and information, and we feel we have either directed them in ways of sorting out possible dietary problems, or else helped them to realize that their problems fall into a different category. I have had to let my personal commitment lapse as I have returned to Health Visiting, and am not available for the sessions. However, I have remained in close contact with them.

As a Group, we have also been asked to give talks locally to other interested organizations. Some of those contacting us recently are the National Childbirth Trust, Local Support Group for Asthma, the National Society for Gifted Children, and the social services department who organise regular speaker sessions. On the day we went along, there were representatives from Child Guidance, Child Psychologists, local Medical Officers and General Practitioners.

Interest in my recipe booklet has continued, and most days I have orders to send off, letters to write to people who have asked for specific information and help or phone calls from those people who prefer to ring and talk.

As I look back over these past few years, we really have had a struggle. I think that one of the most difficult problems is the feeling of total isolation. It is so difficult for people around you to know how you feel. I remember that Rob and I were invited to a dinner party one night. There were eight of us there. We knew two of the other couples very well, but not the third. We were both very tired, and had left our baby sitter, who was well acquainted with the boys, feeling slightly apprehensive, I think. Jeremy was poorly with a chest infection, and the whole house smelt like a chemist's shop, with his vapourisor going in the bedroom. Daniel was coughing, and I knew we would probably be up most of the night with him when we got back. During the evening the conversation turned to family life, and how all our lives had changed fairly dramatically after having children; but that the enjoyment of watching a child grow and develop intellectually, emotionally and physically far outweighed the alterations in social life style. Rob and I listened, but remained fairly passive. Neither of us, if we were totally honest with ourselves, had enjoyed an awful lot of our previous three years. One of the couples whom we didn't know tried to draw us into the conversation, asking about the boys. I remember Robert telling him that we didn't plan fun things to do in advance, because from experience we knew the boys would be ill, or we would be so exhausted we honestly could not be bothered. He told him, "We just try to get through each day." It was quite obvious that the others found this quite unbelievable. Their children were rarely ill. The did not wake up in the mornings until about 7 a.m., and once they were up they were a delight to have around. It is really difficult to understand the experience of the same old weary routine of getting up to very unhappy children, eight, nine, ten times, every night for months on end, if you have rarely had a broken night's sleep yourself. I did not think I would ever forget it, but I must admit the memories are fading now.

Daniel

The older the boys get, the less difficult they are to reason with and to amuse. Their diets are very strictly adhered to. For Daniel, this is an absolute necessity. His physical good health is dependent on meticulous care with his diet, and he has a sound knowledge of exactly what he can and cannot eat. If he isn't sure, he generally refuses it, or comes to ask us. However, there are occasions when he is put very much at risk. On a recent emergency admission to hospital, I found it very difficult to impress on the staff the seriousness of his food allergies, without giving the impression of being an overprotective and anxious mother. In that sort of situation he is extremely vulnerable, and is totally dependent on us, as parents, to ensure that his diet is entirely safe for him. In instances like this it is advisable to cultivate a skin like a rhinoceros! Recently our G.P. suggested that he write a brief letter for us to take away on holiday, in case Daniel needed medical attention. This would reinforce our own explanations.

Jeremy is excellent with his diet. His problems are not so severe, but he knows that he may start to wheeze or get tummy-ache or diarrhoea, if he strays from the straight and narrow. Their social behaviour is quite acceptable to us now, especially when I consider what it used to be like. They are in bed by seven o'clock, and sleep through the night, unless they are wheezing or have an infection which disturbs them. Daniel is still an early riser, waking most mornings between five and six o'clock. He amuses himself far more readily now, doing jig-saws, playing with lego, reading or writing. His brain seems to be on the go from the minute he wakes up. He asks endless questions, and has an insatiable appetite for facts and figures. Both boys have an abundant supply of energy. They are impetuous and impulsive. We have to have eyes in the back of our heads and try to anticipate their every action. I must admit that we still find them very wearing. But they are fit and healthy and physically quite strong. The amount of infections they have requiring antibiotic treatment has very definitely reduced over the last eighteen months.

They have regular dental checks, and their dentist has always been impressed by the quality and soundness of their teeth: even if he does find their excitable behaviour a stark contrast to that of his own two daughters! He is fully aware of their allergic problems, and is meticulously careful to avoid any mouthwashes or pastes which are articifially coloured or flavoured. The boys thoroughly enjoy their visits to him.

Unfortunately, asthma does seem to be becoming more evident. They both now have daily prophylactic treatment. Jeremy has Becotide and Ventolin, and Daniel has Intal, and also needs Ventolin fairly frequently. There is no doubt that wheezing is caused by exercise, infections and many inhalants, as well as food. They take it in good part and both recognise the symptoms and accept the medication readily. Virtually no schooling has been lost through asthma. They do not see wheezing as a "tool" to use against authority, or as an excuse to get out of any particular activity they don't want to do. The only occasions that they possibly recognise that we, as parents, become anxious, is when further medical intervention becomes necessary. Otherwise their wheeze is just a part of them. They both love swimming, and Daniel has recently managed to do his ten metres, on his back and front, without any arm bands. They have also been attending a local "tumble club", another form of physical activity which I feel is good for them, and which they have thoroughly enjoyed.

A great deal more is being understood and published about allergy and food sensitivity. It is an important field of research, and one which I am sure will make many contributions to medicine in the future. I have written this book in response to pressure, initially from friends, and subsequently from many contacts who have suggested it would be helpful and interesting for other families in a similar predicament to read and to identify with. We have been very fortunate in having such excellent support from doctors, family and friends, and although I am quite sure our problems are far from over, we have learnt a lot about ourselves, our inadequacies, our strengths, and weaknesses and we have two lovely boys who look the picture of health, in spite of their problems.

ALLERGY BADGE KIT

1 Cut out or photocopy the following slogans.
2 Colour the background if required.
3 Badge presses can often be found in fairgrounds, shopping arcades etc.

Serious food allergies! Please do not feed me.

I AM VIOLENTLY ALLERGIC TO MANY FOODS

No foods, drinks or sweets please. Severe food allergies!

A FOOD DIARY

A food diary can be very helpful when trying to establish problem foods. It needs to be thorough and carried out for several weeks. Hopefully, some sort of pattern may begin to emerge, e.g. does asthma occur with the same foods such as nuts, or orange juice? Can you link restless, poor nights with any one food or group of foods? Does chocolate produce aggressive, defiant behaviour?

AN EXAMPLE OF A FOOD DIARY

Date	Breakfast	Lunch	Tea	Snack	Comments
1.1.84	Weetabix Sugar Nutramigen	Chicken stew Rhubarb crumble Orange juice	Pate Toast Carob cake	Wholewheat crisps Sesame drops Nutramigen	Diarrhoea
2.1.84	Porridge Syrup Nutramigen	Fish Patties Potato Carrots Treacle tart Pineapple juice	Toast Honey Rice Krispie cake	Cashew nuts Sesame drops Nutramigen	Wheezy Tummy ache
3.1.84	Cornflakes Sugar Nutramigen Toast/honey	Lamb chop Brussel sprouts Potato/gravy Banana Orange juice	Savoury scones Marmite Carob cake Nutramigen	Ginger biscuits Nutramigen	Good day
4.1.84	Porridge Syrup Nutramigen	Spaghetti bolognaise Ground rice with Blackcurrant jelly	Toast Honey Nuts and raisins Rice Krispie cakes	Sesame drops Pineapple juice Crisps	Tummy ache

RECIPE SECTION

I have previously collected together 50 recipes all of which are milk, egg, and additive free. The booklet is called *What Can I give Him Today?*, costs 85p and is available from 19a Parton Rd., Churchdown, Gloucester GL3 2AB.

I have now prepared another recipe section, all new recipes which are simple to make and easy to adapt for individual tastes or needs. Once again I have completely avoided the use of any milk substitute, as this then allows anyone on a cow's milk-free diet to use any of the recipes, without wondering whether their particular milk substitute, be it goat's milk, soya milk or Nutramigen, etc., will alter the texture or taste of any one recipe.

I do use an egg white substitute, which I find makes very acceptable mousse, meringues, macaroons etc., but I have not included any of these recipes, as it is my intention to keep it very simple, and to use only ingredients commonly found in the average pantry. Obviously, margarine has to be bought specially, as normal margarines contain milk products, and usually additives too. I have tried several milk-free margarines, and find the most satisfactory in terms of taste, price and quality in cooking, one obtained from Foodwatch (details in list of addresses). For some children an untreated white flour or stoneground wholemeal flour may be advisable. Be careful of baking powders, as some commercial brands may contain lactose.

As in my previous recipe booklet, my intention has not been to give ideas for main course meals, or a "balanced diet", but to add variety and new ideas for the difficult areas in the child's diet, e.g. snacks, desserts and savoury ideas. From the many letters I have received, the main meals do not provide the problems, but they all say it would be nice to have a new cake recipe to try out, or something different for pudding. I have also been asked, many times, for ideas for babies. Undoubtedly the best milk for a baby is his mother's breast milk. This is of the utmost importance if the baby is born into a family where there is a history of allergy. If, for any reason, the mother is unable, or does not wish, to breast feed, then she must take the advice of her G.P., midwife or Health Visitor, regarding a suitable milk for her infant.

It may be prudent for the breast feeding mother, especially the one who is aware of a family allergy problem, to watch her own diet very carefully, avoiding milk and egg products herself: as long as she does not jeopardise her own nutrition. It certainly would do no harm to avoid the sorts of food and drink which contain artifical additives, and to concentrate on fresh foods, wholefoods, natural fruit juices, etc.

If a baby shows continual signs of possible reactions to his milk, whether it is a cow's milk, formula or breast milk, then medical advice must be sought. In the case of artificially fed infants, a change of milk must only be carried out under medical supervision, as some preparations may be totally unsuitable for a very young baby, and may well place it at risk: in particular, goat's milk and some forms of soya milk fall into this category.

As long as a baby is thriving and content, it is advisable to delay the introduction of weaning foods until the baby is at least four months old, even longer if he is satisfied on his mother's own milk. Foods should then be introduced cautiously, giving only one new taste at a time, and for a few days, in order to see whether the baby has any untoward reaction. A taste of puréed fruit or vegetable is a good starter. If fruits are rather sour and need sweetening, try mixing in a little honey. Never add salt to a young baby's food. When introducing cereals, start with a baby rice, as the wheat-based cereals are common culprits in producing allergic reactions.

Experimenting in providing nourishing, tasty baby meals can be very interesting. Avoid highly spiced items, but otherwise just liquidise a little of your meals, using water or the baby's milk substitute (or breast milk) as the liquid. For example, initially try pureed carrot, or carrot and potato mixed together. When you want to add some protein, try a slice of chicken with the carrot and potato; blend together with chicken stock.

In the initial stages, when only tiny amounts of food are required, try freezing portions in an ice-cube tray. When used they must of course be thoroughly cooked through again.

For desserts, the pureed fruits, such as apple, pear and banana can all be offered, and more "substance" added by mixing in baby rice to thicken. Try making a fresh fruit jelly with gelatin (beware if you are avoiding all beef products as gelatin is made from cow's hide. Foodwatch supply a preservative-free gelatin). Ground rice, mixed with water and flavoured with carob (a cocoa substitute) and natural demerara sugar, makes a nice change. Once a baby is out of the puréed food stage and is eating more textured and substantial meals, then any of the following recipes may be tried.

CONTENTS

A Guide to American Equivalent Weights

Imperial	American
1 lb margarine, or other fat	2 cups
1 lb flour	4 cups
1 lb granulated or castor sugar	2 cups
1 lb brown (moist) sugar	2 cups
12 oz golden syrup	1 cup
8 oz rice	1 cup
5 oz dried fruit	1 cup
1 lb minced meat	2 cups
2 oz soft breadcrumbs	1 cup
½ oz flour	2 tablespoons
1 oz flour	¼ cup
1 oz sugar	2 tablespoons
½ oz margarine	1 tablespoon
1 oz syrup	1 tablespoon

Liquid measures	
¼ pint liquid	⅔ cup
½ pint	1¼ cups
¾ pint	2 cups
1 pint	2½ cups
1½ pints	3¾ cups
2 pints	5 cups

SAVOURY

1. *Chicken Pie*

Ingredients:

6 oz (175 g) shortcrust pastry
½ pint (275 ml) chicken stock
1 oz (25 g) plain flour
1 oz (25 g) margarine

8 oz (225 g) chopped cooked
 chicken
seasoning

Method

Make 6 oz (175 g) short crust pastry, and line the bottom of a pie dish with half of the pastry.

Melt margarine and gradually add flour, cooking gently for one minute. Add chicken stock gradually and bring to the boil. Cook, stirring very carefully, for three minutes. Remove from heat and add chopped chicken and seasoning. Spoon into pie dish, and add the upper pastry crust.

Bake at 400°F (200°C, Gas Mark 6) for 30 minutes. Serve hot or cold.

2. *Chinese Pancakes*

Ingredients:

6 oz (175 g) plain flour
4 fl oz (110 ml) boiling water

salt
oil

Method

Sift flour and salt, pour on boiling water and mix to a manageable dough. If more water is needed, add sparingly. Knead dough until it stretches, elastically. Roll out on floured board to ¾" thick oblong. Cut into even 1" shapes. Take two pieces and flatten each slightly. Smear oil over one side and sandwich two pieces together. Roll out very thinly and roughly circular. Put few drops of oil in flat frying pan and heat to moderate heat. Fry pancake for a minute until light brown underneath. Turn and cook the other side.

suggested filling:

Ingredients:
½ pint (275 ml) chicken stock
1 small onion
1 small potato
¼ lb (110 g) mushrooms
seasoning
tin tuna fish

Method
Cook all ingredients, except tuna fish, in pressure cooker for 5
mins, then liquidize until smooth, thickened sauce. Mash tuna
fish, and add to the sauce. Spread on pancake and roll up.

---

3. *Mincemeat Loaf*

Ingredients:
1 lb (450 g) minced beef
1 small onion
1½ oz (35 g) wholemeal
    breadcrumbs
1 oz (25 g) ground rice
6 tbsps. stock
salt and pepper
1 clove garlic crushed
sprinkle mixed herbs
Worcester Sauce
½ tsp. curry powder

Method
Fry onion lightly in a little oil or milk-free margarine. Blend all
ingredients together in a bowl, mixing thoroughly with fingers.
Mould into a loaf shape: about 3–4" deep and place in a roasting
dish. Cover with foil.

Bake at 375–400°F (190–200°C, Gas Mark 5–6) for about 1 hour.
Remove foil for the last ¼hour.

---

4. *Savoury Scones*

Ingredients:
4 oz (110 g) plain flour
6 oz (175 g) cooked, mashed
    potato
2 tsps. baking powder
½ tsp. mixed herbs
tsp. Worcester Sauce
1½ oz (35 g) milk-free margarine
2 tblsp. water
seasoning

Daniel

Method
Mix flour, baking powder, seasoning and herbs in mixing bowl. Rub in margarine. Add cooked mashed potato, and rub into mixture distributing it well. Add water and Worcester Sauce and mix to a stiff dough. Turn onto floured board, and knead. Roll out to ¾" thick, and cut into rounds.

Bake at 450°F (230°C, Gas Mark 8) for about 12 minutes.

To serve, cut in half and toast under the grill, then spread with home made pate, or marmite.

---

5. Turkey Pate

Ingredients:

4 oz (110 g) cooked turkey
chopped up turkey liver (cooked)
4–5 fluid oz (110–140 ml) turkey gravy or stock

small onion
1 oz (25 g) fresh wholemeal breadcrumbs
seasoning: salt, pepper, pinch mixed herbs

Method
Lightly fry onion. Put all ingredients into liquidizer. Liquidize until smooth consistency. Keep sealed in refrigerator. Excellent for snacks on crispbreads, or on wholemeal baps.

---

6. Fish and Sesame Patties

Ingredients:

12 oz (350 g) cooked flaked fish
12 oz (350 g) cooked potato
½ pint (275 ml) water
1 dessertspoon sesame seeds
½ oz (10 g) milk-free margarine
½ oz (10 g) plain flour

wholemeal breadcrumbs
2 tsp. tomato puree
seasoning:
pinch mixed herbs
salt and pepper
dash of Worcester Sauce

Method
Wash fish, place in a casserole dish with the water and seasoning, and sprinkle the sesame seeds over the contents.

Bake at 375°F (190°C, Gas Mark 5) for ½ hour, or until fish is tender.

Remove from the oven and cool. Cook the potatoes. Flake the fish into a mixing bowl, being careful to remove all bones and skin. Add the cooked potatoes and mash together.

In a saucepan, melt the margarine. Remove from heat, and with wooden spoon, mix in flour. Return to heat and cook for three minutes. Gradually add the fish stock, mixing thoroughly all the time. Cook for further five minutes. Add 2 or 3 tablespoons of this sauce to the fish mixture, to moisten it, and set the rest aside. Then, using your fingers, mould the fish/potato mixture into 12 balls, flatten each one, and coat both sides with breadcrumbs. To the remainder of the sauce add the tomato puree mixing thoroughly, and serve with patties. The patties should be baked for 15 mins. at 400°F (200°C, Gas Mark 6).

---

7. *Potuna Pasties*

Ingredients:

8 oz (225 g) shortcrust pastry	1 tin of tuna fish, flaked
1 small onion	4 small potatoes
1 oz (25 g) margarine	seasoning

Method

Cook potatoes and mash with the margarine and seasoning. Lightly fry the chopped onion and add this to the flaked fish and potato.

Roll out the pastry thinly and using 4½" cutter, cut out six rounds. Pile the mixture over half the circle, moisten edges, and seal the other half pastry over the top of the filling.

Bake at 400°F (200°C, Gas Mark 6) for 20–25 mins.

8. Lentil Soup

Ingredients:

6 oz (175 g) dried lentils
½ oz (10 g) margarine
1 tsp. salt
1 medium onion, finely diced

3 pints (1 litre 750 ml) chicken stock/water
½ oz (10 g) flour
1 bay leaf

Method

Soak the lentils in the stock/water over night. Melt margarine in pressure cooker, stir in flour, add salt, onions bay leaf and lentils with stock. Cook at pressure for 15 mins. Allow cooker to cool slowly. Remove the bay leaf. Place in a blender, for a smooth creamy soup; add a little cooked potato to thicken if necessary, and adjust seasoning.

9. Barbecue Tomato Sauce

This is an excellent sauce accompaniment for either barbecued meals, or served cold with rice and salad.

Ingredients:

1 small onion, finely diced
2–3 tblsp. tomato puree
1 clove garlic crushed
2–3 tblsp. vinegar

6 fl oz (170 ml) fresh pineapple juice
2 tblsp. brown sugar

Method

Put all ingredients into frying pan, bring gently to boil, stirring occasionally. Leave to simmer for 15–20 minutes.

10. *Mushroom Soup*

Ingredients:

¾ pint (425 ml) chicken stock
1 medium onion, peeled and
    chopped
1½ oz (35 g) soft margarine
6 oz (175 g) mushrooms

1 tsp. vecon
1 tsp. marmite
salt/pepper
1 large potato
1 bay leaf

Method
Fry onion until transparent. Wash mushrooms, and cut in half. Put all ingredients into pressure cooker. Cook at 15 lbs pressure for five minutes. Cool, remove bay leaf and liquidize the contents. Serve with a garnish of chopped fresh parsley.

11. *Tomato Sardine Spread*

Ingredients:

1 tin sardines or pilchards in
    tomato sauce
2 oz (50 g) milk-free margarine

2 oz (50 g) soft brown
    breadcrumbs
1 tsp. chopped parsely.

Method
Mash fish well into the tomato sauce. Melt the margarine and mix in the breadcrumbs. Beat mixture all together, and refrigerate. Serve on wholemeal baps.

12. *Herring Roe Paté*

Ingredients:

Herring roe
milk-free margarine

seasoning
Worcester sauce

Method
Lightly fry the roe in the margarine, and allow to cool. Blend with the seasoning and Worcester sauce, and a little margarine. Refrigerate before serving. Serve on crisp brown toast.

93

BISCUITS

13. *Carob Crisps*

Ingredients:
3 oz (75 g) plain flour
1 oz (25 g) cornflour
½ tsp. baking powder
pinch salt

2 oz (50 g) margarine
2 oz (50 g) sugar
1 dessertspoon carob

Method
Rub margarine into flour, cornflour, baking powder and salt. Mix in sugar and carob. Add water to make stiff dough (approx. 2 tblsp. water) Knead lightly. Roll out. Cut into shapes. Bake at 350°F (180°C, Gas Mark 4) for 10 to 15 mins.

14. *Gingerbread Men*

Ingredients:
3 oz (75 g) soft brown sugar
1 tblsp. black treacle
1 tblsp. water
½ tsp. sod. bic.

2 tblsp. golden syrup
3½ oz (90 g) margarine
2 tsps. ground ginger
9 oz (250 g) plain flour

Method
Bring to boiling sugar, syrup, treacle and water, stirring all the time. Remove pan from heat and stir in margarine and bicarbonate of soda. Then stir in flour and ginger to make a smooth dough. More flour may be needed. Rest the dough in refrigerator for 30 mins. Then roll out dough on floured surface, and cut out gingerbread men. Arrange on greased baking sheets.

Bake at 350°F (180°C, Gas Mark 4) for about 10 mins.

15. *Sesame Drops*

Ingredients:
3 oz (75 g) margarine
2 oz (50 g) sugar   4 oz (110 g) s.r. flour
sesame seeds   1 tsp. water

Method
Cream butter, sugar and water. Sieve flour, add to the creamed mixture, binding together. Roll into small balls and dip one side into sesame seeds. Flatten slightly on greased trays (sesame seeds uppermost). These biscuits flatten during cooking.

Bake at 375°F (190°C, Gas Mark 5) for about 12 mins.

16. *Ginger Biscuits*

Ingredients:
4 oz (110 g) margarine   1 tblsp. syrup
1 pinch bicarbonate of soda   1 tsp. ground ginger
6 oz (175 g) flour   3 oz (75 g) castor sugar

Method
Melt margarine and golden syrup and stir in rest of ingredients. Put teaspoonsful onto greased trays.

Bake at 375°F (190°C, Gas Mark 5) for 10 mins.

17. *Lemon Crunch Slices*

Ingredients:
6 oz (175 g) margarine   3 oz (75 g) castor sugar
4 oz (110 g) coconut   6 oz (175 g) s.r. flour
2 oz (50 g) cornflakes   grated rind of 1 lemon

Method
Grease and line Swiss roll tin. Melt margarine and sugar gently in saucepan. Leave to cool. In a bowl mix flour and coconut. Stir in

warmed mixture and mix well together. Fold in cornflakes and lemon rind. Press evenly into tin.

Bake at 350°F (180°C, Gas Mark 4) for 30–35 mins. Firm to touch and light golden. Cut while warm.

---

18. *Oatmeal Biscuits*

Ingredients:

4 oz (110 g) s.r. flour   ½ tsp. salt
4 oz (110 g) rolled oats   2 oz (50 g) castor sugar
3 oz (75 g) black treacle   4 oz (110 g) margarine

Method
Sieve flour and salt. Stir in rolled oats, melt sugar, black treacle and margarine. Add to the dry ingredients. Press into a greased Swiss roll tin. Sprinkle with coarse oatmeal.

Bake at 350°F (180°C, Gas Mark 4) for 20–25 mins.

---

19. *Oat Drops*

Ingredients:

5 oz (150 g) s.r. flour   3 oz (75 g) oats
3 oz (75 g) sugar   ½ tsp. bicarbonate soda
2 oz (50 g) margarine   2 oz (50 g) lard.
1 tblsp. golden syrup

Method
In a saucepan, melt margarine, lard and golden syrup. In a bowl thoroughly mix all dry ingredients. Add melted mixture to dry ingredients and blend together well. Form into balls, place on greased tray.

Bake at 350°F (180°C, Gas Mark 4) for 15 minutes.

20. *Ginger Crunch*

Ingredients:

2 oz (50 g) margarine	2 level tblsp. syrup
3 oz (75 g) s.r. flour	½ tsp. ground ginger
1 oz (25 g) castor sugar	2 oz (50 g) Rice Krispies

Method

Melt margarine and syrup over low heat. Mix all dry ingredients in bowl. Add the melted mixture and mix thoroughly. Press into Swiss Roll tin.

Bake at 350°F (180°C, Gas Mark 4) for 12–13 mins.

21. *Viennese Sandwich Biscuit*

Ingredients:

6 oz (175 g) margarine	6 oz (175 g) s.r. flour
2 oz (50 g) castor sugar	

Method

Cream the fat and sugar. Thoroughly mix in the sifted flour. Either pipe onto greased baking sheets, or drop spoonfuls onto the sheet.

Bake at 325–350°F (170–180°C, Gas Mark 3–4) for 20–25 mins.

Sandwich with jam and butter cream.

22. *Mixibiscs.*

Ingredients:

4 oz (110 g) margarine	2 oz (50 g) porridge oats
3 oz (75 g) brown sugar	1 oz (25 g) chopped nuts
1 tblsp. syrup	½ oz (10 g) sesame seeds
4 oz (110 g) s.r. flour	½ oz (10 g) raisins

Method

Heat the margarine, sugar and syrup in a pan. Mix the remaining ingredients in a bowl. Add the melted mixture. Mix well.

Bake at 325°F (170°C, Gas Mark 3) 12– 15 mins.

23. *Peanut Shortbread*

Ingredients:
4 oz (110 g) salted peanuts
4 oz (110 g) s.r. flour
5 oz (150 g) plain flour

3 oz (75 g) brown sugar
6 oz (175 g) margarine

Method
Wash and dry peanuts. Scatter over base of a Swiss roll tin. Rub margarine into dry ingredients until mixture resembles bread-crumbs. Pour these on top of the nuts and gently press the mixture into the tin with your knuckles.

Bake at 375°F (190°C, Gas Mark 5) for 25–30 mins. Cut into fingers while warm, but allow to cool in the tin, before turning out, upside down onto a cooling rack.

DESSERTS

24. *Treacle and Ground Rice Tart*

Ingredients:

4 oz (110 g) shortcrust pastry
2 tblsp. golden syrup
½ oz (10 g) margarine

1 oz (25 g) ground rice
1 oz (25 g) wholemeal
    breadcrumbs

Method

Line a flan dish. In a saucepan melt syrup and margarine. Remove from heat and add rice and breadcrumbs. Mix together thoroughly, and spoon into pastry case.

Bake at 375°F (190°C, Gas Mark 5) for 25 mins.

25. *Banana Crunch*

Ingredients:

6 oz (175 g) margarine
6 oz (175 g) s.r. flour
6 oz (175 g) semolina

3 oz (75 g) castor sugar
2 bananas

Method

Heat margarine in large pan. Remove from heat, stir in flour, semolina and sugar. Lightly grease Swiss roll tin, and spread half mixture over base of tin. Press firmly. Slice bananas over top and put rest of mixture on top.

Bake at 400°F (200°C, Gas Mark 6) for 30 mins. Leave in tin to cool. Cut into fingers.

26. *Rhubarb and Honey Crumble Crunch*

Ingredients:

1 lb (450 g) rhubarb
1 tblsp. honey
2 tblsp. water
4 oz (110 g) wholewheat flour
2½ oz (60 g) margarine

3 oz (75 g) natural demerara
  sugar
2 oz (50 g) wholewheat
  breadcrumbs
1 oz (25 g) coconut

Method

Wash and clean the rhubarb and cut into 1″ pieces. Place in bottom of oven proof dish, dot with the honey and add about 3 tblsps. water.

Rub margarine into flour, add sugar, breadcrumbs and coconut and mix thoroughly, spoon over the rhubarb.

Bake at 375°F (190°C, Gas Mark 5) for about 1 hour.

27. *Rhubarb Flan*

Ingredients:

6 oz (175 g) McVities Digestive
  biscuits
3 oz (75 g) milk-free margarine
2 oz (50 g) brown sugar

1 lb (450 g) rhubarb
castor sugar to sweeten
1 dessertspoon golden syrup

Method

Place biscuits in a polythene bag and crush a with rolling pin. Melt the margarine and syrup in a saucepan, slowly. Remove from heat. Add sugar and crushed biscuits. Mix well, then press firmly into a flan dish, to cover base and sides. Lightly cook rhubarb, sweeten to taste. Put into liquidizer, straining off at least half of the juice. Pour liquidized mixture into flan case. Serve chilled.

28. *Blackcurrant and Pear Flan*

Ingredients:
4 oz (110 g) plain flour
pinch salt
2 oz (50 g) lard
water to mix
3 dessert pears

¼ pint (150 ml) water
1 level tsp. gelatine
2 heaped dessertsp. blackcurrant
   jelly

Method

Rub together flour, salt and lard. Mix with about 2 tblsp. cold water to a firm dough. Roll out onto floured board and line a flan case. Bake at 400°F (200°C, Gas Mark 6) for 25 mins.

Peel, core and slice pears into the base of the flan case. Blend the gelatine into cold water, put into the saucepan with the blackcurrant jelly and bring slowly to the boil, stirring all the time. Cook gently for 5 mins. Cool and pour over pears. Serve chilled.

29. *Caramelled Pears*

Ingredients:
3 oz (75 g) castor sugar
7 fl oz (200 ml) water
4 firm pears

Method

Stir the sugar and half the water in a saucepan, until the sugar has dissolved, then boil until golden brown. Add the rest of the water. Stir over a low heat until you have a pouring sauce. Peel, core and slice pears. Put them into the caramel and cook for about 10 mins. Serve sprinkled with chopped nuts and raisins if permitted.

30. *Rhubarb Sponge Pudding*

Ingredients:

Approx. 6 sticks rhubarb
4 oz (110 g) plain flour
1½ oz (35 g) margarine
2 oz (50 g) sugar

pinch salt
½ tsp. baking powder
water

Method

Wash and slice the rhubarb into a pie dish. Rub margarine into the dry ingredients. Mix to a moist dough with water and spread evenly over the rhubarb. Bake at 375°F (190°C, Gas Mark 5) for 25 mins.

CAKES

31. *Ginger Sponge*

Ingredients:

4 oz (110 g) margarine
5 fl oz (140 ml) water
1 level tsp. bicarbonate of soda
4 oz (110 g) castor sugar

3 level tblsp. golden syrup
8 oz (225 g) s.r. flour
2 level tsp. ground ginger

Method
Grease and line 7 x 11 x 1¼" tin

Melt margarine, syrup and water in saucepan. Into a bowl, sift flour, bicarbonate of soda, and ginger. Stir in sugar. Make well in middle, and pour in syrup mixture. Beat with wooden spoon until smooth. Pour into tin.

Bake at 325°F (170°C, Gas Mark 3) for 35 mins. or until firm and springy. Cool in tin, then cut into squares.

32. *Banana Scone*

Ingredients:

8 oz (225 g) s.r. flour
2 level tsp. baking powder
¼ level teasp. salt
2 oz (50 g) margarine

½ lb (225 g) bananas, peeled and mashed
2 oz (50 g) demerara sugar
4 tblsp. water

Method
Sift flour, salt and baking powder into bowl. Rub in margarine; stir in mashed banana and sugar and enough water to give a soft manageable dough. Knead on floured surface and cut into a circle about ¾" thick. Mark 8 wedges. Bake at 425°F (220°C, Gas Mark 7) for about 20 mins.

---

33. *"Chocolate" Buns*

Ingredients:

8 oz (225 g) plain flour
4 oz (110 g) sugar
1 tsp. baking powder
3 oz (75 g) margarine
pinch salt

water
Sauce filling:
2 level tbsp. golden syrup
1 heaped tsp. carob

Method

Rub margarine into dry ingredients. Mix to stiff dough with water. Put balls of dough into paper cases, in bun trays. Make a hole in top of each bun.

Melt syrup and carob in saucepan. With a teaspoon pour a little of this mixture into each bun.

Bake at 325°F (170°C, Gas Mark 3) for 12–15 mins.

---

34. *"Chocolate" Cake*

Ingredients:

10 oz (275 g) s.r. flour
4½ oz (125 g) margarine
2 tsps. carob

5 oz (150 g) castor sugar
6 fl oz (170 ml) water
1 tsp. bicarbonate soda

Method

Mix flour and sugar together in bowl. Rub in margarine. In saucepan heat water; add carob and bicarbonate of soda. When frothy, add to rubbed in mixture. Mix with wooden spoon, thoroughly. Divide into two 7″ sandwich tins, greased and lined.

Bake at 325°F (170°C, Gas Mark 3) for 30 mins.

35. *Banana Cake*

Ingredients:

12 oz (350 g) plain flour
1 tsp. salt
4 oz (110 g) margarine
2 large bananas

3 tsps. baking powder
¼ tsp. bicarbonate soda
8 oz (225 g) castor sugar
4 fl oz (110 ml) water

Method

Cream margarine and sugar until light and fluffy. Add water gradually, beating very well. Sift all dry ingredients together and add alternately with mashed bananas. Blend well together. Pour into two 8″ sandwich tins, greased and lined.

Bake at 375°F (190°C, Gas Mark 5) for 30 mins.

36. *Coconut Ring*

Ingredients:

4 oz (110 g) coconut
6 oz (175 g) castor sugar
8 oz (225 g) s.r. flour
4 oz (110 g) margarine

1 tsp. baking powder
6 fl oz (170 ml) warm water
1 tsp. bicarbonate of soda

Method

Grease a 9″ ring mould, very thoroughly.

Cream margarine and sugar. Mix bicarbonate of soda into the water. Mix the sifted dry ingredients alternately with the liquid. Beat well until blended. Spoon into ring mould.

Bake at 350°F (180°C, Gas Mark 4) for approx. 40 mins. Turn out immediately.

37. *Jam Sponge Tarts*

Ingredients:
4 oz (110 g) shortcrust pastry

Method
Roll out and cut with pastry cutter. Line jam tart tins.

Sponge mixture
2 oz (50 g) margarine	½ level tsp. bicarbonate soda
1 tblsp. syrup	2 oz (50 g) castor sugar
2 fl oz (60 ml) boiling water	jam
4 oz (110 g) s.r. flour	

Method
Melt the margarine, syrup and boiling water together in a saucepan. Mix dry ingredients in a bowl. Add melted mixture to them and mix thoroughly. Put a teaspoonful of favourite jam into each pastry case, and a dessertspoonful of sponge mixture on top of this. Bake for 25 mins., or until firm and springy , at 375°F (190°C, Gas Mark 5).

38. *Carrot and Cinnamon Cake*

Ingredients:
8 oz (225 g) plain flour	4 oz (110 g) margarine
pinch salt	4 oz (110 g) honey
1 dessertspoon cinammon	4 oz (110 g) brown sugar
½ tblsp. bicarbonate of soda	8 oz (225 g) grated carrot
1 tsp. nutmeg	

Method
Mix together in a bowl flour, salt, cinnamon, bicarbonate of soda and nutmeg. In a saucepan melt the margarine, honey and brown sugar. Add this to the dry ingredients. Mix the grated carrot into the mixture last of all. Spoon into a greased and lined loaf tin. Bake at 325°F (170°C, Gas Mark 3) for 1 hour.

39. *Banana Cream Cake*

Ingredients:

8 oz (225 g) s.r. flour
6 oz (175 g) castor sugar
2 tsps. baking powder
½ tsp. bicarbonate of soda

4 oz (110 g) margarine
2 large ripe bananas
Approx. 2 fl oz (60 ml) water

Method

Sift all dry ingredients into large bowl. In another bowl blend the margarine and bananas together. Add to the dry ingredients, mixing with a little water until well blended. Pour into two 8″ sandwich tins (greased and lined).

Bake at 375°F (190°C, Gas Mark 5) for 25–30 mins. Cool for 10 mins. then turn out onto wire rack. Sandwich with buttercream icing.

PRESERVES

40. *Rhubarb Jam*

Ingredients:
1 lb (450 g) freshly cut rhubarb
1 lb (450 g) sugar
1 tblsp. water

Method
Clean and cut the rhubarb into small pieces. Put into saucepan with water, and slowly bring to boil. When rhubarb is cooked and soft add sugar and boil rapidly until set is obtained: approx 20 mins.

41. *Blackcurrant Jelly*

Ingredients:
2 lb (900 g) blackcurrants
1 pint (570 ml) water
sugar

Method
Simmer fruit until very soft. (Pressure cook at 15 lbs pressure for 5 mins.) Strain through a muslin or a jelly bag, overnight. Repeat above procedure, this time simmering the pulp that is left in a further ½ pint water (285 ml). Strain through jelly bag, into original juice. Measure juice. Allow 1 lb (450 g) sugar to each pint (570 ml) of juice. Stir in sugar, and boil rapidly until set.

42. *Rhubarb and Lemon Jam*

Ingredients:
3 lb (1 kg 350 g) rhubarb
3 large lemons
3 lb (1 kg 350 g) sugar

Method
Slice the rhubarb into small pieces and put into a large bowl, with layers of sugar. Add juice of 3 lemons. Cover and leave overnight.

Put into saucepan, and add the grated rind of two of the lemons. Bring to the boil, and boil rapidly until set.

43. *Rosehip Syrup*

Ingredients:
2 lb (900 g) ripe rose hips
4½ pints (2 litres 555 ml) water
1 lb (450 g) sugar

Method
Coarsely mince, grate or chop the ripe rose hips. Add to 3 pints (1 litre 710 ml) of briskly boiling water. Return to the boil. Remove pan from the heat. Leave to stand for 10 mins. Drip through jelly bag. Put pulp back into saucepan, and add a further 1½ pints (845 ml) water. Bring to the boil, then leave for a further 10 minutes. Strain through jelly bag, once more into first batch of juice. Pour into the pan, and boil rapidly until liquid has reduced to ¾ pint. (425 ml) Add sugar, stirring over low heat until dissolved. Pour into screw top bottles, leaving about 1" headroom. Screw on tops, then loosen by ¼ turn. Stand bottles in a deep pan of cold water, on a rack. Slowly bring water to simmering, and continue to simmer for 20 mins. Carefully remove bottles, and stand them on a wooden surface. Tighten screw tops and label.

Dilute with water to serve.

44. *Rhubarb Chutney*

Ingredients:

1 lb (450 g) onions, finely
    chopped
½ pint (275 ml) vinegar
3 lbs (1 kg 350 g) rhubarb

1 tsp. pickling spice
1 tsp. salt
1 tsp. ground ginger
12 oz (350 g) sugar

Method

Put onions, rhubarb, pickling spices (tied securely in muslin), salt, and ginger into pressure cooker, with the vinegar. Cook at 15 lbs pressure for 5 mins. Cool slowly. Add sugar, stirring carefully. Boil steadily until the chutney is thick. Remove pickling spices. Pour into hot jars.

DOUGHS AND PASTRY

45. *Sweet Buns*

Ingredients:

1 lb 10 oz (750 g) strong white
 flour
½ tsp. salt
2 oz (50 g) butter
2 tblsp. castor sugar
2 oz (50 g) mixed fruit (optional)
1 tblsp. sesame seeds

½ oz (10 g) fresh yeast
16 fl oz (455 ml) warm water
Glaze
1 tblsp. sugar
2 tblsp. hot water
sesame seeds

Method

Mix yeast with tsp. sugar and a little of warm water. Leave it in a warm place to froth.

Sift flour and salt into large bowl. Rub in margarine. Add sugar, sesame seeds, and fruit if desired.

Add yeast and water and mix thoroughly into mixture. Knead on lightly floured board. Return to oiled bowl, and leave to double its size. (cover bowl with oiled cling film)

Make glaze by dissolving sugar in water. Cut dough into approx. 16 pieces. Knead each piece separately. Shape into round. Brush with glaze, and scatter top of each bun with sesame seeds. Place on greased baking tray. Leave to rise until double in size. Cover with cling film.

Bake at 425°F (220°C, Gas Mark 7) for 10 mins. Delicious spread with margarine and rhubarb jam!

46. Brown Baps

Ingredients:
13 oz (375 g) strong white flour
½ tsp. salt
½ (10 g) fresh yeast

13 oz (375 g) wholewheat flour
2 oz (50 g) milk-free margarine
16 fl oz (455 ml) warm water

Method
This recipe makes a plain version of the preceding buns. Use entirely the same method. Sesame seeds or carraway seeds may be used, by using a glaze and sprinkling on top, if liked. They certainly add a crunchy texture, as well as an interesting flavour.

47. Wholemeal Pastry

Ingredients:
6 oz (175 g) wholemeal flour
3 oz (75 g) milk-free margarine
½ tsp. salt

Method
Mix flour and salt in bowl. Cut margarine into pieces, and rub into flour.

Add 2 tblsp. water to this mixture, and stir with knife. Then still in bowl, knead it together gently until a firm dough. This is then easier to handle, if left in a polythene bag in fridge, for 15 mins.

Bake at 400°F (200°C, Gas Mark 6) for 20–30 mins, according to nature of recipe.

48. Ruff Puff Pastry

Ingredients:
8 oz (225 g) s.r. flour
5 oz (150 g) lard (or lard and
  margarine)

½ tsp. salt
Approx. ¼ pint (150 ml) cold
  water

Method

Mix flour and salt in basin, add the fat cut into small pieces. Stir them in with a knife. Mix to a stiff paste with the water. Turn onto a floured board. Roll into a narrow strip. Fold this into three, turn one of the open sides towards you, and roll out again. Do this three times. Leave the pastry to rest, then roll into the shape desired.

49. *Jam Squares*

8 oz (225 g) Ruff Puff pastry rolled out to about ¼". Using a square pastry cutter, cut out an even number of squares. Using a small round cutter (e.g. a bottle top) cut the centre out of half of the squares. Damp the edges, and place one of the "holey" squares on top of a complete square.

Bake at 400°F (200°C, Gas Mark 6) for 15 mins. Fill the holes with favourite jam. Serve fresh.

50. *Currant Slices*

8 oz (225 g) Ruff Puff pastry rolled out into two equal size oblongs. Lightly cover one of these with a little favourite jam. Scatter currants or mixed dried fruit over and dot with tiny pieces of margarine. Place other oblong on the top, sealing the edges. Sprinkle with sugar. Bake at 400°F (200°C, Gas Mark 6) for 20 mins. Cut into fingers when cool. Serve fresh.

IDEAS FOR PACKED LUNCHES

Sandwich fillings: Variety can be obtained by using white or wholemeal bread, baps or crispbreads.

Home-made paté fish or meat

Marmite

honey

Sardine in tomato sauce

roast chicken with home-made stuffing

tuna: mashed with knob of margarine, seasoned with herbs, salt and pepper or Worcester sauce.

peanut butter

home-made jam: rhubarb, blackcurrant jelly, pineapple

Savoury tartlets made with ruff puff or shortcrust pastry and filled with meat paté, a fishy mixture (tuna, sardine, herring roe) or a savoury chicken mixture.

Cold chicken drum sticks.

Sausages on sticks. Many butchers, if requested, will make up sausage recipes to specific instructions, if you are able to buy a sensible quantity and freeze them. These may also be used for sausage rolls, again using either ruff puff or shortcrust pastry. Bulk buying with friends also makes this more worthwhile for the butcher.

Crisps: Some supermarkets produce their own brand of ready salted crisps, which are free from all additives. Whole food stores also stock wheat crisps, made from natural products.

Nuts and raisins. Cashew nuts.

Salad snacks individually packed, containing grated carrot, radish, cucumber, celery, cold potato etc.

Home-made soups, stored in wide-necked flasks, are easy to eat with a spoon. Team this up with a wholemeal bap.

Permitted fruit or individually packed fruit salad.

Home-made cake and biscuits.

There are now a variety of commercially produced "natural" confectionery bars, which are milk, egg and additive free. Look out for sesame snack biscuits, a nutritious snack.

Drinks: There are a variety of pure fruit juices on the market now, which clearly state that they are free from artificial additives, and preservatives. They may be used diluted, to help them go further. At least one firm is now producing pure fruit

114

syrups, which can be used as fruit drinks, or to flavour mousses, desserts etc.

One firm also makes additive-free orange and lemon squash, and this is becoming available in many supermarkets.

Hot savoury drinks may be made from marmite or vecon (a natural vegetable stock).

All children enjoy eating sweets. Unfortunately, the vast majority of commercial confectionary contains large quantities of artificial colour and flavours. Some chemists stock quality sweets made from natural colours and flavours, not always expensive. There are a variety of "spangle" type boiled sweets which retail at 14p per packet. The secret is always to have an eye on ingredients labelling.

"Foodwatch" supply sticks of rock made from natural ingredients, also a variety of boiled sweets. Mint imperials are usually additive free.

Glossary of Medical Terms Used in the Book

Allergen A substance that stimulates a harmful reaction in the body, known as allergy

Allergy The body's reaction to a foreign substance which is normally harmless

Analgesia Pain relieving medicine

Anaphylactic reaction A severe, immediate reaction that calls for emergency treatment

Antibody A protein produced by the body to fight foreign materials that enter it. Another name for antibodies is immunoglobulins: normally shortened to Ig's.

Bricanyl A drug used to relieve bronchospasm

Colostrum The first fluid produced by the breasts after childbirth

Conjunctivitis Inflammation of the mucous membrane covering the eyeball

Hydrocortisone A steroid which suppresses an inflammatory reaction

Hypoglycaemia Lowering of the blood sugar level

Infantile eczema An inflammatory condition of the skin which is non-contagious and very itchy

Intal Sodium Cromoglycate. A drug given to prevent asthmatic attacks. It is inhaled, and therefore works directly on the lungs

Immune System The body's natural defense mechanism protecting the individual against disease and infection

Nalcrom Sodium Cromoglycate. A drug given to help prevent allergic reactions in the gut. It is taken orally.

Nutramigen A hydrolysed casein feed containing sucrose and corn oil, used in the management of infants and children sensitive to whole protein. Only to be used when directed by your doctor.

Nebulized Ventolin A method of giving Ventolin (a drug which relieves bronchospasm) by inhalation through a mask held to the face.

Oedema Swelling into the tissues.

Oilatum   An arachis oil preparation used in scaling disorders, where a cleansing agent is required which is not irritant to the skin

Paediatrician   A specialist in the diseases of children

Piriton   An anti-allergic drug containing an antihistamine

Pneumo-mediastinum   Air in the cavity which surrounds the heart, leaking from a hole in the lung

Salicylate   Literally, a salt of salicylic acid. Salicylates are found naturally in many fruits and a few vegetables: such as blackberries, raspberries, strawberries, apples, plums and tomatoes. Aspirin is a compound of salicylic acid.

Stapphyloccus   A bacteria, often pus-producing, which attacks and infects skin

Streptococcus   A bacteria often responsible for causing acute ear and throat infections

Urticaria   Nettle-rash, or hives. A skin condition characterized by the recurrent appearance of an eruption of weals, causing great irritation.

Addresses and Useful Organizations

1 Hyperactive Children's Support Group (HACSG)
  Mrs. Sally Bunday (Secretary)
  59, Meadowside,
  Angmering,
  West Sussex
  BN16 4BW

2 Foodwatch,
  Butts Pond Industrial Estate,
  Stourminister Newton,
  Dorset
  DT10 1AZ

3 Eczema Society
  Tavistock House North,
  Tavistock Square,
  London WC1H 9SR

4 Action Against Allergy,
  43, The Downs,
  London S.W.20

USEFUL BOOKS

Parents Book of Childhood Allergies, Richard F. Graber, Ballatine Books

Parents' Guide to Allergy in Children, Claude Frazier M.D., Grosset & Dunlap, 1978

Coping and Living with Allergies, Claude Frazier M.D., Spectrum

The Hyperactive Child, Belinda Barnes & Irene Coluhoun, Thorsons Publishing Group

What Can I Give Him Today?, Diana Wells, (50 milk, egg, additive free recipes), 85p., available from 19a Parton Rd., Churchdown, Gloucester GL3 2AB

Parties Make Me Sick, Rae Paterson & Judy McKechnie, Alma Publications, Australia. A story for and about children who have problems with food

Food For Thought, A Parents' Guide to Food Intolerance, Maureen Minchin, Alma Publications and George Allen & Unwin, Australia